3 Keys To Managing

PTSD

THE WARRIOR'S GUIDE TO OVERCOMING COMBAT TRAUMA

WORKBOOK EDITION

BRETT COTTER

ISBN: 978-0-9965029-2-4

www.StressIsGone.org

Dedication

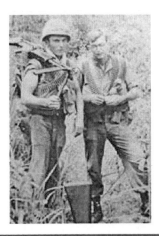 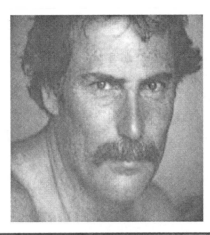 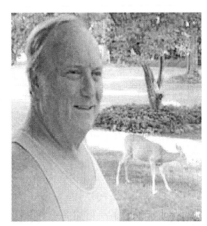

This book is dedicated to a proud father of five who died from long-term complications from PTSD. A man who endured a very rough life, yet despite regrets, entertained everyone he met.

He rode Harley's, played ball, lived fast, did it all. He sang in street corner bands and built buildings with his bare hands. Funny beyond words can say, belly laughs left ribs hurting the next day. He lived outside the boundaries most of us know; great jokes ready to go, he always put on a really good show.

He was encouraging and kind, and brave and out of his mind. The strongest, the funniest, yet humble beyond compare. I learned of his feats with my own eyes and from his brothers, when he was no longer there. It was never a competition, he included everyone in his fun crazy mission.

Later his priorities changed. Family relationships once strained; where mended and remained. He could sense my bad day; he would call and know exactly what to say. A lasting message he sent, "Amazing things happen when you're in the moment."

A decorated New York City Firefighter with Ladder 30 and Rescue 3; decorated Marine Vietnam Veteran M60 Machine Gunner who served with C Co. / 2nd Bn. / 7th Mar. / 1st Mar. Div. participating in Operations: Golden Fleece, Perry, Union II, Arizona, Sierra, Rio Grand and Brown.

He could fix everything, do anything, but he couldn't slow down. This book is dedicated to Cpl John J. Cotter, Jr. 2/22/1948 - 10/09/2014. I know you're having fun up there. Thanks for motivating me to write this book. **I love you Dad.**

Preface

50% of those with PTSD do not seek treatment. (Tanielian and Jaycox, 2008)

This book is for anyone who wants to naturally reduce their stress levels.

I was coaching an OEF-A veteran who was diagnosed with PTSD. He called me just after he had an auto accident. A car struck his vehicle from the side. When the police officer arrived, the other driver started blaming the accident on the veteran. The police officer started to believe the other driver's story. As I'm hearing this, I'm getting concerned because it sounded like a situation that would trigger an intense PTSD reaction. So I asked him what happened and he said, "I know the program is working, because after we all drove off, I realized I was calm the entire time."

There are multiple generations of combat veterans in my family. I have seen first-hand how PTSD can affect a person and their loved ones. Given my 15-year career in stress management; teaching corporate classes, providing one-on-one coaching, and creating the Stress Is Gone Method, I wanted to share the tools I've seen work time and time again.

The program you will learn is certified by The American Institute of Stress. This book is a great tool, however, you're going on a mission. Successful missions require a good team using the right tools. The goal of this mission is to return your life back to its natural state, before the trauma occurred. This is not a solo mission. I want you to call-in for backup and have your team at your fingertips, to assist whenever you like. Your team includes family, friends, healthcare professionals, etc. As you know, with a good team and the right tools, any mission is possible. You are in command.

Read *3 Keys to Managing PTSD* thoroughly. This book will help you sleep at night, gain more control in stressful situations, learn how to meditate and will help you process traumatic memories.

As you read on, please keep in mind that I am not a scientist or a clinician. I am a stress relief expert. This is not written for the *Wall Street Journal*, it's for The Warrior.

The hardest part is over; you already lived through it. Now it's time to learn how to let go mentally, physically, and emotionally.

Introduction

Post-Traumatic Stress affects approximately 7.7 million American adults each year. Everyday 22 veterans commit suicide. Former Defense Secretary Leon Panetta referred to this as an "epidemic". Vietnam veterans with PTSD are more than twice as likely to develop heart disease. Iraq and Afghanistan veterans with PTSD symptoms are three times more likely to report suicidal thoughts and hopelessness.

As a stress relief expert who coaches people with PTSD, *The Warrior's Guide* lays out 3 essential keys that have been helping my clients. Now, I share this information with you.

The 3 keys are:

(1) Learn how to stop a stress reaction
(2) Process the trauma
(3) Meditate daily

The 3 keys are explained in depth, providing you with easy-to-follow exercises to master each key.

This book provides a fresh new look at PTSD and discusses some of the complexities combat veterans face. A step-by-step roadmap is clearly laid out to help anyone interested in decreasing stress levels.

You are further supported by a free mobile app and complimentary online resources to help predict stress, shut down reactions, process trauma, and meditate everyday.

"As a Doctor of 14 years, prior service member, and Director for a Civilian Navy SEAL Training Program, I understand stress. Stress Is Gone uses unique and innovative ways to help those seeking to manage emotional stressors. I have found their approach to be helpful with my patients overall sense of wellness and use the Stress Is Gone Program daily in my practice." ~ **Dr. Stephen M. Erle**

I will make you the same promise I make to everyone in my class; *"If you follow these exercises 100%, I guarantee, you will release more stress today than you ever have in your entire life."* ~ **Brett Cotter**

Table of Contents

Chapter 1: What Is PTSD?

If we compare our body's typical fight-or-flight reaction to a handgun, then PTSD is more like a machine gun.

Introduction

Stressful memories do not just disappear over time; they sub-consciously accumulate and affect our behavior. PTSD is the brain's way of venting the accumulated stress from traumatic events that were never processed.

The Basics

When a person experiences a life-and-death event and does not fully process the trauma (mentally, emotionally, and physically), the brain uses secondary outlets to systematically vent the accumulated stress. Secondary outlets are flashbacks, nightmares, and displaced triggers.

Displaced triggers are circumstances that trigger a PTSD reaction. For example; unexpected loud noises, interacting with authority figures, being around large crowds, having to wait in lines or in traffic, challenging dynamics at home or in the workplace, or any situation that feels out of one's control. When secondary outlets trigger a PTSD reaction, the person feels as if they are in a survival situation, even though there is no immediate life-and-death threat.

Simply put, PTSD is like comparing a basic handgun (typical fight-or-flight reaction) to the M60 Machine Gun (PTSD survival reaction). Now imagine that M60 has a very sensitive trigger, is in full automatic mode, and has a misaligned targeting system. Firing a weapon like that could leave even an expert marksman feeling confused, overwhelmed, depressed and have devastating effects on oneself and others. PTSD weakens areas of our life in which we've previously known success, connection, confidence, and clarity.

Summary

PTSD is the brain's way of venting accumulated unprocessed trauma through displaced triggers, flashbacks, and nightmares.

Chapter 2: Understanding PTSD

The deeper we understand a problem the more we can affect it.

Introduction

There are 3 core complexities that make PTSD very unique and difficult to manage. Understanding these complexities will help us properly address them. This chapter also includes the *PTSD Score Card*, which enables you to track your progress over the next twelve months.

A Deeper Look

- *Hyper-Alert*: Combat training rewires our *fight-or-flight* reaction to *kill-or-be killed*. This resets a person's nervous system to be hyper-alert, which results in frequent overreactions. This re-programming helps us survive combat, but greatly complicates civilian life.

- *Adrenaline Overload*: The adrenalin of combat fries our central nervous system. Humans are not designed to endure survival situations for long periods of time. Imagine filling up a 1957 Chevy with nitrous oxide and racing cross-country. And if you were fortunate enough to reach the finish line, you were then expected to drive slowly, in the same car, with the same fuel, for the rest of your life.

- *Trauma Buildup*: The immense amount of life-and-death trauma a combat veteran experiences accumulates below the surface and impacts the ability to clearly perceive and respond in the environment. Even though a traumatic memory may not be in the forefront of one's thoughts, the experience effects everyday functioning. Up to 90% of our mental processing occurs on the unconscious level.

Symptoms

PTSD symptoms can appear months or years after a traumatic event. Exercise 2.1 shows a list of symptoms. Circle your score for symptom frequency (how often it occurs) and intensity. Add the subtotals at the bottom of the page to generate your symptom score. Exercise 2.1 is repeated 12 times for 1 year of use. Rescore your symptoms once a month to stay aware of your overall stress levels, recognize which symptoms are reducing, and be mindful of new symptoms on the rise. If you are consistently using the tools in this book you can expect your score to lower over time. Only score symptoms you experience. This is not a diagnostic tool; it's part of your stress management plan. (chapter continues on page 15)

Exercise 2.1 (1) PTSD Score Card   **Date: ___/___/_____**

Physical Symptoms	Frequency			Intensity		
	Mthly	**Weekly**	**Daily**	**Low**	**Mid**	**High**
Headaches / Migraines	1	2	3	1	2	3
Dizziness	1	2	3	1	2	3
Fatigue	1	2	3	1	2	3
Chest Pain	1	2	3	1	2	3
Breathing Difficulties	1	2	3	1	2	3
Stomach / Digestive Issues	1	2	3	1	2	3
Subtotals =	(	)		(	)	

Psychological Symptoms	Frequency			Intensity		
	Mthly	**Weekly**	**Daily**	**Low**	**Mid**	**High**
Depression	1	2	3	1	2	3
Low Self Esteem	1	2	3	1	2	3
Feeling Hopeless	1	2	3	1	2	3
Anxiety	1	2	3	1	2	3
Guilt / Survivor's Guilt	1	2	3	1	2	3
Lack of Emotion	1	2	3	1	2	3
Flashbacks	1	2	3	1	2	3
Hallucinations	1	2	3	1	2	3
Subtotals =	(	)		(	)	

Behavioral Symptoms	Frequency			Intensity		
	Mthly	**Weekly**	**Daily**	**Low**	**Mid**	**High**
Extreme Rage	1	2	3	1	2	3
Short Fuse	1	2	3	1	2	3
Isolating	1	2	3	1	2	3
Alcohol / Drug Abuse	1	2	3	1	2	3
Self Medicating	1	2	3	1	2	3
Always on Guard	1	2	3	1	2	3
Easily Startled	1	2	3	1	2	3
Feeling Numb	1	2	3	1	2	3
Lack of Concentration	1	2	3	1	2	3
Memory Issues	1	2	3	1	2	3
Nightmares	1	2	3	1	2	3
Unable to Sleep Soundly	1	2	3	1	2	3
Hopeless About Future	1	2	3	1	2	3
Lack of Appetite	1	2	3	1	2	3
Overeating	1	2	3	1	2	3
Subtotals =	(	)		(	)	

Total Score (add all subtotals for one overall score) =

Exercise 2.1 (2) PTSD Score Card   **Date:** ___/___/_____

Physical Symptoms		Frequency			Intensity	
	Mthly	Weekly	Daily	Low	Mid	High
Headaches / Migraines	1	2	3	1	2	3
Dizziness	1	2	3	1	2	3
Fatigue	1	2	3	1	2	3
Chest Pain	1	2	3	1	2	3
Breathing Difficulties	1	2	3	1	2	3
Stomach / Digestive Issues	1	2	3	1	2	3
Subtotals =		(	)		(	)

Psychological Symptoms		Frequency			Intensity	
	Mthly	Weekly	Daily	Low	Mid	High
Depression	1	2	3	1	2	3
Low Self Esteem	1	2	3	1	2	3
Feeling Hopeless	1	2	3	1	2	3
Anxiety	1	2	3	1	2	3
Guilt / Survivor's Guilt	1	2	3	1	2	3
Lack of Emotion	1	2	3	1	2	3
Flashbacks	1	2	3	1	2	3
Hallucinations	1	2	3	1	2	3
Subtotals =		(	)		(	)

Behavioral Symptoms		Frequency			Intensity	
	Mthly	Weekly	Daily	Low	Mid	High
Extreme Rage	1	2	3	1	2	3
Short Fuse	1	2	3	1	2	3
Isolating	1	2	3	1	2	3
Alcohol / Drug Abuse	1	2	3	1	2	3
Self Medicating	1	2	3	1	2	3
Always on Guard	1	2	3	1	2	3
Easily Startled	1	2	3	1	2	3
Feeling Numb	1	2	3	1	2	3
Lack of Concentration	1	2	3	1	2	3
Memory Issues	1	2	3	1	2	3
Nightmares	1	2	3	1	2	3
Unable to Sleep Soundly	1	2	3	1	2	3
Hopeless About Future	1	2	3	1	2	3
Lack of Appetite	1	2	3	1	2	3
Overeating	1	2	3	1	2	3
Subtotals =		(	)		(	)

Total Score (add all subtotals for one overall score) =

Exercise 2.1 (3) PTSD Score Card   Date: ___/___/_____

Physical Symptoms	Frequency			Intensity		
	Mthly	_Weekly_	_Daily_	_Low_	_Mid_	_High_
Headaches / Migraines	1	2	3	1	2	3
Dizziness	1	2	3	1	2	3
Fatigue	1	2	3	1	2	3
Chest Pain	1	2	3	1	2	3
Breathing Difficulties	1	2	3	1	2	3
Stomach / Digestive Issues	1	2	3	1	2	3
Subtotals =		(	)		(	)

Psychological Symptoms	Frequency			Intensity		
	Mthly	_Weekly_	_Daily_	_Low_	_Mid_	_High_
Depression	1	2	3	1	2	3
Low Self Esteem	1	2	3	1	2	3
Feeling Hopeless	1	2	3	1	2	3
Anxiety	1	2	3	1	2	3
Guilt / Survivor's Guilt	1	2	3	1	2	3
Lack of Emotion	1	2	3	1	2	3
Flashbacks	1	2	3	1	2	3
Hallucinations	1	2	3	1	2	3
Subtotals =		(	)		(	)

Behavioral Symptoms	Frequency			Intensity		
	Mthly	_Weekly_	_Daily_	_Low_	_Mid_	_High_
Extreme Rage	1	2	3	1	2	3
Short Fuse	1	2	3	1	2	3
Isolating	1	2	3	1	2	3
Alcohol / Drug Abuse	1	2	3	1	2	3
Self Medicating	1	2	3	1	2	3
Always on Guard	1	2	3	1	2	3
Easily Startled	1	2	3	1	2	3
Feeling Numb	1	2	3	1	2	3
Lack of Concentration	1	2	3	1	2	3
Memory Issues	1	2	3	1	2	3
Nightmares	1	2	3	1	2	3
Unable to Sleep Soundly	1	2	3	1	2	3
Hopeless About Future	1	2	3	1	2	3
Lack of Appetite	1	2	3	1	2	3
Overeating	1	2	3	1	2	3
Subtotals =		(	)		(	)

Total Score (add all subtotals for one overall score) =

Exercise 2.1 (4) PTSD Score Card   Date: ___/___/_____

Physical Symptoms	Frequency			Intensity		
	Mthly	*Weekly*	*Daily*	*Low*	*Mid*	*High*
Headaches / Migraines	1	2	3	1	2	3
Dizziness	1	2	3	1	2	3
Fatigue	1	2	3	1	2	3
Chest Pain	1	2	3	1	2	3
Breathing Difficulties	1	2	3	1	2	3
Stomach / Digestive Issues	1	2	3	1	2	3
Subtotals =	(	)		(	)	

Psychological Symptoms	Frequency			Intensity		
	Mthly	*Weekly*	*Daily*	*Low*	*Mid*	*High*
Depression	1	2	3	1	2	3
Low Self Esteem	1	2	3	1	2	3
Feeling Hopeless	1	2	3	1	2	3
Anxiety	1	2	3	1	2	3
Guilt / Survivor's Guilt	1	2	3	1	2	3
Lack of Emotion	1	2	3	1	2	3
Flashbacks	1	2	3	1	2	3
Hallucinations	1	2	3	1	2	3
Subtotals =	(	)		(	)	

Behavioral Symptoms	Frequency			Intensity		
	Mthly	*Weekly*	*Daily*	*Low*	*Mid*	*High*
Extreme Rage	1	2	3	1	2	3
Short Fuse	1	2	3	1	2	3
Isolating	1	2	3	1	2	3
Alcohol / Drug Abuse	1	2	3	1	2	3
Self Medicating	1	2	3	1	2	3
Always on Guard	1	2	3	1	2	3
Easily Startled	1	2	3	1	2	3
Feeling Numb	1	2	3	1	2	3
Lack of Concentration	1	2	3	1	2	3
Memory Issues	1	2	3	1	2	3
Nightmares	1	2	3	1	2	3
Unable to Sleep Soundly	1	2	3	1	2	3
Hopeless About Future	1	2	3	1	2	3
Lack of Appetite	1	2	3	1	2	3
Overeating	1	2	3	1	2	3
Subtotals =	(	)		(	)	

Total Score (add all subtotals for one overall score) =

Exercise 2.1 (5) PTSD Score Card   Date: ___/___/_____

Physical Symptoms	**Mthly**	Frequency **Weekly**	**Daily**	**Low**	Intensity **Mid**	**High**
Headaches / Migraines	1	2	3	1	2	3
Dizziness	1	2	3	1	2	3
Fatigue	1	2	3	1	2	3
Chest Pain	1	2	3	1	2	3
Breathing Difficulties	1	2	3	1	2	3
Stomach / Digestive Issues	1	2	3	1	2	3
Subtotals =		( )			( )	

Psychological Symptoms	**Mthly**	Frequency **Weekly**	**Daily**	**Low**	Intensity **Mid**	**High**
Depression	1	2	3	1	2	3
Low Self Esteem	1	2	3	1	2	3
Feeling Hopeless	1	2	3	1	2	3
Anxiety	1	2	3	1	2	3
Guilt / Survivor's Guilt	1	2	3	1	2	3
Lack of Emotion	1	2	3	1	2	3
Flashbacks	1	2	3	1	2	3
Hallucinations	1	2	3	1	2	3
Subtotals =		( )			( )	

Behavioral Symptoms	**Mthly**	Frequency **Weekly**	**Daily**	**Low**	Intensity **Mid**	**High**
Extreme Rage	1	2	3	1	2	3
Short Fuse	1	2	3	1	2	3
Isolating	1	2	3	1	2	3
Alcohol / Drug Abuse	1	2	3	1	2	3
Self Medicating	1	2	3	1	2	3
Always on Guard	1	2	3	1	2	3
Easily Startled	1	2	3	1	2	3
Feeling Numb	1	2	3	1	2	3
Lack of Concentration	1	2	3	1	2	3
Memory Issues	1	2	3	1	2	3
Nightmares	1	2	3	1	2	3
Unable to Sleep Soundly	1	2	3	1	2	3
Hopeless About Future	1	2	3	1	2	3
Lack of Appetite	1	2	3	1	2	3
Overeating	1	2	3	1	2	3
Subtotals =		( )			( )	

Total Score (add all subtotals for one overall score) =

Exercise 2.1 (6) PTSD Score Card Date: ___/___/_____

Physical Symptoms	Frequency			Intensity		
	Mthly	Weekly	Daily	Low	Mid	High
Headaches / Migraines	1	2	3	1	2	3
Dizziness	1	2	3	1	2	3
Fatigue	1	2	3	1	2	3
Chest Pain	1	2	3	1	2	3
Breathing Difficulties	1	2	3	1	2	3
Stomach / Digestive Issues	1	2	3	1	2	3
Subtotals =	(	)		(	)	

Psychological Symptoms	Frequency			Intensity		
	Mthly	Weekly	Daily	Low	Mid	High
Depression	1	2	3	1	2	3
Low Self Esteem	1	2	3	1	2	3
Feeling Hopeless	1	2	3	1	2	3
Anxiety	1	2	3	1	2	3
Guilt / Survivor's Guilt	1	2	3	1	2	3
Lack of Emotion	1	2	3	1	2	3
Flashbacks	1	2	3	1	2	3
Hallucinations	1	2	3	1	2	3
Subtotals =	(	)		(	)	

Behavioral Symptoms	Frequency			Intensity		
	Mthly	Weekly	Daily	Low	Mid	High
Extreme Rage	1	2	3	1	2	3
Short Fuse	1	2	3	1	2	3
Isolating	1	2	3	1	2	3
Alcohol / Drug Abuse	1	2	3	1	2	3
Self Medicating	1	2	3	1	2	3
Always on Guard	1	2	3	1	2	3
Easily Startled	1	2	3	1	2	3
Feeling Numb	1	2	3	1	2	3
Lack of Concentration	1	2	3	1	2	3
Memory Issues	1	2	3	1	2	3
Nightmares	1	2	3	1	2	3
Unable to Sleep Soundly	1	2	3	1	2	3
Hopeless About Future	1	2	3	1	2	3
Lack of Appetite	1	2	3	1	2	3
Overeating	1	2	3	1	2	3
Subtotals =	(	)		(	)	

Total Score (add all subtotals for one overall score) =

Exercise 2.1 (7) PTSD Score Card　　　　　　　Date: ___/___/_____

Physical Symptoms	Frequency			Intensity		
	Mthly	Weekly	Daily	Low	Mid	High
Headaches / Migraines	1	2	3	1	2	3
Dizziness	1	2	3	1	2	3
Fatigue	1	2	3	1	2	3
Chest Pain	1	2	3	1	2	3
Breathing Difficulties	1	2	3	1	2	3
Stomach / Digestive Issues	1	2	3	1	2	3
Subtotals =	(	)		(	)	

Psychological Symptoms	Frequency			Intensity		
	Mthly	Weekly	Daily	Low	Mid	High
Depression	1	2	3	1	2	3
Low Self Esteem	1	2	3	1	2	3
Feeling Hopeless	1	2	3	1	2	3
Anxiety	1	2	3	1	2	3
Guilt / Survivor's Guilt	1	2	3	1	2	3
Lack of Emotion	1	2	3	1	2	3
Flashbacks	1	2	3	1	2	3
Hallucinations	1	2	3	1	2	3
Subtotals =	(	)		(	)	

Behavioral Symptoms	Frequency			Intensity		
	Mthly	Weekly	Daily	Low	Mid	High
Extreme Rage	1	2	3	1	2	3
Short Fuse	1	2	3	1	2	3
Isolating	1	2	3	1	2	3
Alcohol / Drug Abuse	1	2	3	1	2	3
Self Medicating	1	2	3	1	2	3
Always on Guard	1	2	3	1	2	3
Easily Startled	1	2	3	1	2	3
Feeling Numb	1	2	3	1	2	3
Lack of Concentration	1	2	3	1	2	3
Memory Issues	1	2	3	1	2	3
Nightmares	1	2	3	1	2	3
Unable to Sleep Soundly	1	2	3	1	2	3
Hopeless About Future	1	2	3	1	2	3
Lack of Appetite	1	2	3	1	2	3
Overeating	1	2	3	1	2	3
Subtotals =	(	)		(	)	

Total Score (add all subtotals for one overall score) =

Exercise 2.1 (8) PTSD Score Card   Date: ___/___/_____

Physical Symptoms	Frequency			Intensity		
	Mthly	_Weekly_	_Daily_	_Low_	_Mid_	_High_
Headaches / Migraines	1	2	3	1	2	3
Dizziness	1	2	3	1	2	3
Fatigue	1	2	3	1	2	3
Chest Pain	1	2	3	1	2	3
Breathing Difficulties	1	2	3	1	2	3
Stomach / Digestive Issues	1	2	3	1	2	3
Subtotals =	(	)		(	)	

Psychological Symptoms	Frequency			Intensity		
	Mthly	_Weekly_	_Daily_	_Low_	_Mid_	_High_
Depression	1	2	3	1	2	3
Low Self Esteem	1	2	3	1	2	3
Feeling Hopeless	1	2	3	1	2	3
Anxiety	1	2	3	1	2	3
Guilt / Survivor's Guilt	1	2	3	1	2	3
Lack of Emotion	1	2	3	1	2	3
Flashbacks	1	2	3	1	2	3
Hallucinations	1	2	3	1	2	3
Subtotals =	(	)		(	)	

Behavioral Symptoms	Frequency			Intensity		
	Mthly	_Weekly_	_Daily_	_Low_	_Mid_	_High_
Extreme Rage	1	2	3	1	2	3
Short Fuse	1	2	3	1	2	3
Isolating	1	2	3	1	2	3
Alcohol / Drug Abuse	1	2	3	1	2	3
Self Medicating	1	2	3	1	2	3
Always on Guard	1	2	3	1	2	3
Easily Startled	1	2	3	1	2	3
Feeling Numb	1	2	3	1	2	3
Lack of Concentration	1	2	3	1	2	3
Memory Issues	1	2	3	1	2	3
Nightmares	1	2	3	1	2	3
Unable to Sleep Soundly	1	2	3	1	2	3
Hopeless About Future	1	2	3	1	2	3
Lack of Appetite	1	2	3	1	2	3
Overeating	1	2	3	1	2	3
Subtotals =	(	)		(	)	

Total Score (add all subtotals for one overall score) =

Exercise 2.1 (9) PTSD Score Card   Date: ___/___/_____

Physical Symptoms	Frequency			Intensity		
	Mthly	**Weekly**	**Daily**	**Low**	**Mid**	**High**
Headaches / Migraines	1	2	3	1	2	3
Dizziness	1	2	3	1	2	3
Fatigue	1	2	3	1	2	3
Chest Pain	1	2	3	1	2	3
Breathing Difficulties	1	2	3	1	2	3
Stomach / Digestive Issues	1	2	3	1	2	3
Subtotals =	(	)		(	)	

Psychological Symptoms	Frequency			Intensity		
	Mthly	**Weekly**	**Daily**	**Low**	**Mid**	**High**
Depression	1	2	3	1	2	3
Low Self Esteem	1	2	3	1	2	3
Feeling Hopeless	1	2	3	1	2	3
Anxiety	1	2	3	1	2	3
Guilt / Survivor's Guilt	1	2	3	1	2	3
Lack of Emotion	1	2	3	1	2	3
Flashbacks	1	2	3	1	2	3
Hallucinations	1	2	3	1	2	3
Subtotals =	(	)		(	)	

Behavioral Symptoms	Frequency			Intensity		
	Mthly	**Weekly**	**Daily**	**Low**	**Mid**	**High**
Extreme Rage	1	2	3	1	2	3
Short Fuse	1	2	3	1	2	3
Isolating	1	2	3	1	2	3
Alcohol / Drug Abuse	1	2	3	1	2	3
Self Medicating	1	2	3	1	2	3
Always on Guard	1	2	3	1	2	3
Easily Startled	1	2	3	1	2	3
Feeling Numb	1	2	3	1	2	3
Lack of Concentration	1	2	3	1	2	3
Memory Issues	1	2	3	1	2	3
Nightmares	1	2	3	1	2	3
Unable to Sleep Soundly	1	2	3	1	2	3
Hopeless About Future	1	2	3	1	2	3
Lack of Appetite	1	2	3	1	2	3
Overeating	1	2	3	1	2	3
Subtotals =	(	)		(	)	

Total Score (add all subtotals for one overall score) =

Exercise 2.1 (10) PTSD Score Card   Date: ___/___/_____

Physical Symptoms	Frequency			Intensity		
	Mthly	_Weekly_	_Daily_	_Low_	_Mid_	_High_
Headaches / Migraines	1	2	3	1	2	3
Dizziness	1	2	3	1	2	3
Fatigue	1	2	3	1	2	3
Chest Pain	1	2	3	1	2	3
Breathing Difficulties	1	2	3	1	2	3
Stomach / Digestive Issues	1	2	3	1	2	3
Subtotals =	(	)		(	)	

Psychological Symptoms	Frequency			Intensity		
	Mthly	_Weekly_	_Daily_	_Low_	_Mid_	_High_
Depression	1	2	3	1	2	3
Low Self Esteem	1	2	3	1	2	3
Feeling Hopeless	1	2	3	1	2	3
Anxiety	1	2	3	1	2	3
Guilt / Survivor's Guilt	1	2	3	1	2	3
Lack of Emotion	1	2	3	1	2	3
Flashbacks	1	2	3	1	2	3
Hallucinations	1	2	3	1	2	3
Subtotals =	(	)		(	)	

Behavioral Symptoms	Frequency			Intensity		
	Mthly	_Weekly_	_Daily_	_Low_	_Mid_	_High_
Extreme Rage	1	2	3	1	2	3
Short Fuse	1	2	3	1	2	3
Isolating	1	2	3	1	2	3
Alcohol / Drug Abuse	1	2	3	1	2	3
Self Medicating	1	2	3	1	2	3
Always on Guard	1	2	3	1	2	3
Easily Startled	1	2	3	1	2	3
Feeling Numb	1	2	3	1	2	3
Lack of Concentration	1	2	3	1	2	3
Memory Issues	1	2	3	1	2	3
Nightmares	1	2	3	1	2	3
Unable to Sleep Soundly	1	2	3	1	2	3
Hopeless About Future	1	2	3	1	2	3
Lack of Appetite	1	2	3	1	2	3
Overeating	1	2	3	1	2	3
Subtotals =	(	)		(	)	

Total Score (add all subtotals for one overall score) =

Exercise 2.1 (11) PTSD Score Card Date: ___/___/_____

Physical Symptoms	Frequency			Intensity		
	Mthly	_Weekly_	_Daily_	_Low_	_Mid_	_High_
Headaches / Migraines	1	2	3	1	2	3
Dizziness	1	2	3	1	2	3
Fatigue	1	2	3	1	2	3
Chest Pain	1	2	3	1	2	3
Breathing Difficulties	1	2	3	1	2	3
Stomach / Digestive Issues	1	2	3	1	2	3
Subtotals =	(	)		(	)	

Psychological Symptoms	Frequency			Intensity		
	Mthly	_Weekly_	_Daily_	_Low_	_Mid_	_High_
Depression	1	2	3	1	2	3
Low Self Esteem	1	2	3	1	2	3
Feeling Hopeless	1	2	3	1	2	3
Anxiety	1	2	3	1	2	3
Guilt / Survivor's Guilt	1	2	3	1	2	3
Lack of Emotion	1	2	3	1	2	3
Flashbacks	1	2	3	1	2	3
Hallucinations	1	2	3	1	2	3
Subtotals =	(	)		(	)	

Behavioral Symptoms	Frequency			Intensity		
	Mthly	_Weekly_	_Daily_	_Low_	_Mid_	_High_
Extreme Rage	1	2	3	1	2	3
Short Fuse	1	2	3	1	2	3
Isolating	1	2	3	1	2	3
Alcohol / Drug Abuse	1	2	3	1	2	3
Self Medicating	1	2	3	1	2	3
Always on Guard	1	2	3	1	2	3
Easily Startled	1	2	3	1	2	3
Feeling Numb	1	2	3	1	2	3
Lack of Concentration	1	2	3	1	2	3
Memory Issues	1	2	3	1	2	3
Nightmares	1	2	3	1	2	3
Unable to Sleep Soundly	1	2	3	1	2	3
Hopeless About Future	1	2	3	1	2	3
Lack of Appetite	1	2	3	1	2	3
Overeating	1	2	3	1	2	3
Subtotals =	(	)		(	)	

Total Score (add all subtotals for one overall score) =

Exercise 2.1 (12) PTSD Score Card   Date: ___/___/_____

Physical Symptoms	Frequency			Intensity		
	Mthly	*Weekly*	*Daily*	*Low*	*Mid*	*High*
Headaches / Migraines	1	2	3	1	2	3
Dizziness	1	2	3	1	2	3
Fatigue	1	2	3	1	2	3
Chest Pain	1	2	3	1	2	3
Breathing Difficulties	1	2	3	1	2	3
Stomach / Digestive Issues	1	2	3	1	2	3
Subtotals =	(	)		(	)	

Psychological Symptoms	Frequency			Intensity		
	Mthly	*Weekly*	*Daily*	*Low*	*Mid*	*High*
Depression	1	2	3	1	2	3
Low Self Esteem	1	2	3	1	2	3
Feeling Hopeless	1	2	3	1	2	3
Anxiety	1	2	3	1	2	3
Guilt / Survivor's Guilt	1	2	3	1	2	3
Lack of Emotion	1	2	3	1	2	3
Flashbacks	1	2	3	1	2	3
Hallucinations	1	2	3	1	2	3
Subtotals =	(	)		(	)	

Behavioral Symptoms	Frequency			Intensity		
	Mthly	*Weekly*	*Daily*	*Low*	*Mid*	*High*
Extreme Rage	1	2	3	1	2	3
Short Fuse	1	2	3	1	2	3
Isolating	1	2	3	1	2	3
Alcohol / Drug Abuse	1	2	3	1	2	3
Self Medicating	1	2	3	1	2	3
Always on Guard	1	2	3	1	2	3
Easily Startled	1	2	3	1	2	3
Feeling Numb	1	2	3	1	2	3
Lack of Concentration	1	2	3	1	2	3
Memory Issues	1	2	3	1	2	3
Nightmares	1	2	3	1	2	3
Unable to Sleep Soundly	1	2	3	1	2	3
Hopeless About Future	1	2	3	1	2	3
Lack of Appetite	1	2	3	1	2	3
Overeating	1	2	3	1	2	3
Subtotals =	(	)		(	)	

Total Score (add all subtotals for one overall score) =

It's imperative to stay aware of your symptoms and how efficiently you are managing them. If left unmanaged, PTSD results in a rapidly over firing fight-or-flight reaction. This causes serious health issues, which could have been prevented, such as heart disease, liver disease, autoimmune disease, diabetes, arthritis, obesity, high blood pressure, irritable bowel syndrome, interstitial cystitis, chronic fatigue, fibromyalgia, stomach aches, constipation, body aches and pain, chronic headaches and migraines.

Summary

The hyper-alertness, adrenaline overload, and trauma buildup from combat training and combat experience changes how our brain perceives and responds to danger. It's irrational to expect the central nervous system to function naturally after such experiences.

To minimize future health risks stemming from PTSD, be aware of your symptoms and use the tools in this book to reduce their frequency and intensity.

"This program and mobile app have helped me manage my PTSD symptoms and reminds me to meditate daily. The app guides me through the techniques that are easy to practice anywhere, at anytime. My overall stress level is much less and I am able to handle high stress situations more clearly. I recommend the program to anyone suffering from PTSD."

~ Kyle, Veteran, Southbury, Connecticut

"Stress Is Gone uses easy steps to help readers work through Post Traumatic Stress (PTS) with a proven technique and user friendly program. If you're trying to learn how to manage your stress, the PTSD FREE mobile app is a great addition to your relaxation and meditation program. I would absolutely recommend using Stress Is Gone to help manage your PTS symptoms."

~Juliet Madsen, US Army Retired
Founder, www.strokeofluckquilting.com

Chapter 3: The 1ˢᵗ Key –
Learn How to Stop a Stress Reaction

Unmanaged stress reactions are a more dangerous risk factor for cancer and heart disease than cigarettes or high cholesterol foods. (Cryer, 1996)

Once we realize the reaction, we can side-step the stress.

Introduction

Our cells want to let go of stress. When any living organism on this planet becomes stressed, it's pre-programmed to return to homeostasis as quickly as possible. So, our cells really want to let go of stress and become calm again. Because we are not taught how to effectively process stress, our mind inhibits the body's natural ability to let go. Our mind attaches to stress, and we get caught in mental loops of repeating stressful thoughts stemming from the past or worrisome thoughts about the future.

We'll discuss how to focus your mind and your body at the same time, to let go.

Before we can stop a reaction, we must learn how to recognize when our body is stressed real-time. Here are four Stress Signals to look out for that will help you *realize the reaction.* The moment you see one of these stress signals, a little light bulb should flash on inside your head as you tell yourself, "Oh yeah, my body is stressed again."

Stress Signals

1. *Breath Rate (respiration rate)* - Taking short shallow breaths is a definite sign that your body is stressed. Pay attention to how you are breathing throughout your day. When you realize your breaths are short and shallow tell yourself, "Oh yeah, my body is stressed again."

2. *Heart Rate* – Your heart rate is your body's **[Check Engine]** light. Pay attention to it. When your heart starts pounding, that's your body sounding the alarm, telling you there's a problem. When you realize your heart rate is extra fast tell yourself, "Oh yeah, my body is stressed again."

3. *Mental State* – Whenever you find yourself repeating the same stressful thought, such as: "I gotta get out of here," "I can't take it anymore," "this shouldn't be happening to me," etc. I want you to tell yourself, "Oh yeah, my body is stressed again."

4. *Emotional State* – Whenever you find yourself feeling angry, sad, overwhelmed, jealous, upset, etc. I want you to tell yourself, "Oh yeah, my body is stressed again."

Stress Awareness

Once you realized your body is stressed I want you to observe the reaction. This will help you side-step the stress. Here are three simple tips:

(a) Listen to your thoughts like you're listening to the radio.

(b) Watch the tension build in your body like you're watching T.V.

(c) Identify with the part of yourself that is observing the reaction, not the part reacting.

Methodology - Stopping a Stress Reaction

Now that you are able to realize your reaction and observe it, it's time to learn how to stop a stress reaction.

The fight-or-flight reaction is physiologically responsible for all the stress we experience. The 3 steps described in Exercise 3.1 disengage the fight-or-flight reaction by quickly activating the body's relaxation response. This new technique is named Stress Stopper Breathwork and is certified by The American Institute of Stress. Practice now for 5 minutes.

Exercise 3.1 Stress Stopper Breathwork

Step 1 - Touch the Tension. Gently place your hand on the area that is tense when you are stressed (usually the chest, stomach, or head). Touch is therapeutic. The calm cells in your hand help the tense cells in your body return to homeostasis, a stable state of being. This begins to physically disengage stress.

Step 2 - Breathe Deep and Slow. Science proves breathing deep and slow helps us manually shift gears from stressed to rest. This transfers control from your sympathetic nervous system (which manages stress) to your parasympathetic nervous system (which manages rest). This begins to emotionally disengage stress.

Step 3 - Once per breath, silently say, "I'm Okay". Mantras, similar to autosuggestion or self-hypnosis, have been used to elicit deep relaxation for thousands of years. The "I'm Okay" mantra is the reverse logic that drives our *fight-or-flight reaction*, which is, "I must run or fight to stay alive." This begins to mentally disengage stress.

Practice

Do your best to remain aware of your Stress Signals, and practice Stress Stopper Breathwork throughout your day. In the beginning, it may take a few minutes to realize the reaction. Over time you will recognize your stress signals quicker and increase your daily *stress awareness*. Your goal is to become *stress smart*, and in time you will.

Practice *Stress Stopper Breathwork* every time you become stressed. This is an internal technique that can be done clandestinely wherever you are. Also, practice for 5 minutes when you first wake up in the morning and when you go to sleep at night. Consistent practice helps your body and mind assimilate with the technique, so when you need real-time relief, your body will respond quickly.

If you have trouble falling asleep at night, keep a pen and pad next to your bed. Just before turning off the lights, write out your recurring thoughts and worries. Then turn the page over and write down three very simple actions you can take the next day to address those worries. Look at what you wrote. Turn off the lights and use Stress Stopper Breathwork to fall asleep.

Your three actions should be easy to do. For example, if you are worried that you need to find a job, your actions might be:

1. Look for a job online for 15-minutes,
2. Review my resume,
3. Prepare my best interview attire.

Our brain automatically keeps us awake when it's concerned for our wellbeing. When we write out our biggest worries and three simple solutions, our brain sees we are aware of the problem and that we are addressing it. This stops our brain from unconsciously worrying and lets us rest.

If you wake up in the middle of the night, do not turn on the TV or get up. Keep your eyes closed and practice Stress Stopper Breathwork until you fall back asleep.

Summary

Initially, it may take 5 minutes for Stress Stopper Breathwork to shut down your reaction. Within one month of consistent practice, your mind and body assimilate with the technique, empowering you to stop stress in seconds. Eventually you will be so in-tune with your body, you'll be able to sense your stressor coming around the corner, and use the technique to remain calm when it shows up.

Chapter 4: The 2nd Key – Process the Trauma

60% of men and 50% of women experience some type of trauma in their lifetime. (Norris and Slone, 2013)

We cannot change a past event in history, but we can change the emotions imprinted on the memory.

This chapter helps you process the traumatic memories that fuel PTSD reactions. While working with these memories, it's important to have your team a phone call away. Your team includes people you trust. Those you can rely on and talk to whenever you want support. This may include family members, friends, healthcare professionals, etc. Make a list of contacts below and keep it handy.

MY TEAM

Name:_____   Phone:_____

Name:_____   Phone:_____

Name:_____   Phone:_____

Name:_____   Phone:_____

Name:_____   Phone:_____

Name:_____   Phone:_____

Name:_____   Phone:_____

Introduction

The technique we'll use to process trauma is based on observations, inferences, and practices I have used throughout my 15-year career as a stress relief coach. Let's discuss a few concepts to lay the groundwork for a deeper discussion:

Consistent relaxation accelerates relief. Without conscious effort, our cells process emotional trauma slowly. As life goes on, traumas accumulate and negatively affect the functioning of our central nervous system. If a person never receives help to process traumatic events, the memories sit subconsciously and cause us to overreact.

We need to incorporate routine relaxation into our daily life to assist our body's natural ability to process trauma and regularly restore our nervous system. Daily use of Stress Stopper Breathwork, meditation, restorative yoga, yoga nidra, etc. are examples of techniques you can use to consistently relax. The true key is relaxing the emotions connected to the traumatic memory.

Our brain is in constant contact with our body. Have you ever wondered why our body experiences stress if we merely think about something stressful? Our brain automatically and continuously sends messages to our cells about each thought and perception we have. Similar to the NEWS ticker that scrolls across the bottom of the TV screen, you can imagine these messages as a constant flow of mental status updates from our brain to our body.

Our cells have limited comprehension. Have you ever wondered why we feel stress in our body if we think about a past stressful event? If we know the event is over, why is our fight-or-flight being triggered? And why does stress trigger if we worry about the future? Why is our body freaking out about something that has not even happened?

Our cells don't understand the concept of past and future. Every status update from the brain registers in the body as a real-time message for the present moment. Whether it's a stressful memory from our past or a worry about the future, our body protects itself in the present moment. Furthermore, our cells cannot tell the difference between what is seen in reality and what is imagined mentally. This is why our body experiences stress, when we close our eyes and imagine a stressful event, even one that has never actually happened to us (i.e. if we imagine being chased by a bear in the woods).

Methodology – Process the Trauma

Traumatic memories are at the root of PTSD. These memories are imprinted with the emotional tension experienced during the traumatic event. Each time a PTSD reaction is triggered, these same feelings flare up again and again. We cannot change a past event in history, but we can process the emotional imprint on the memory to a more balanced state. Remember, our cells can't distinguish between past, present, or future. They experience everything as the present moment.

You will learn how to use your body's relaxation response to naturally process traumatic memories. You will saturate these memories with relaxation until they reframe in your psyche. The bulk of your PTSD reactions are usually fueled by a few core traumatic memories. As each core traumatic memory is processed, PTSD symptoms reduce.

While completing Exercise 4.1, write your answers in the space provided next to the questions. Focus on one trigger and one memory at a time. You can also conduct this exercise by using the *Resolve tab* on the *PTSD FREE* mobile app and on the *Stress Is Gone Membership Website*. Both are free resources accessible on the Stress Is Gone website (www.StressIsGone.org) by clicking the *Free Military Veterans Account* icon on the bottom left side of the page. If you prefer writing your answers into this workbook, Exercise 4.1 is repeated 12 times so you can experience 12 separate sessions. If you feel this exercise is helping, I recommend doing it one to four times a month, until you are satisfied with your overall stress level.

Exercise 4.1 will help you:

(1) Assess your most frequent *PTSD reactions*,
(2) Identify which memories are fueling those reactions, and
(3) Process the trauma imprinted on those memories.

(chapter continues on page 70)

Exercise 4.1 (1) Process the Trauma   **Date:** ___/___/_____

Give yourself at least 50 minutes of undisturbed space, have your team a phone call away for support, and see the process to the end.

Step 1. Routine PTSD Assessment

Assess your most frequent PTSD reaction by answering the below questions;

(a) What is the one thing that triggers your PTSD reactions most often?

_____

_____

_____

(b) Where are you when this reaction is most often triggered?

_____

_____

_____

(c) What time of day and which days of the week is this reaction most likely to occur?

_____

_____

_____

(d) Which emotion is predominant during this PTSD reaction?

_____

_____

_____

(e) What thought repeats in your head during this PTSD reaction?

_____

_____

_____

(f) Where do you feel tension right now while thinking about this reaction?

_____

_____

_____

Step 2. Repressed PTSD Assessment

Look back on your life. Identify which memory is fueling this PTSD reaction by answering the below questions;

(g) What is the 1st time you can remember thinking (insert answer from (e) here)

_____

_____

_____

and feeling (insert answer from (d) here) _____

_____

_____

_____

at the same time?

_____

_____

_____

(h) Who or what caused that previous stress reaction?

_____

_____

_____

(i) Where do you feel tension in your body while thinking about this memory?

_____

_____

_____

Step 3. Process the Trauma

Use Stress Stopper Breathwork to release tension from the traumatic memory by following the below steps;

(j) Lie down, close your eyes, and for two minutes breathe deep and slow with your right hand on your (insert answer from (f) here) _____

_____

_____

_____

and your left hand on your (insert answer from (i) here) _____

_____

_____

_____

Once per breath, silently say, "I'm okay".

(k) Think of the memory involving (insert answer from (h) here) _____

_____

_____

_____

(l) Observe your body's reaction as you let the memory play out to a stressful moment. Then pause the memory.

(m) Imagine yourself inside that memory calmly saying, "I'm okay", once per breath, as you continually breathe deep and slow with two hands gently resting where you feel tension in your body.

Continue Step (m) for 20 minutes or until you feel the tension release from your body and from the memory. Waves of emotions will come and go. Continually focusing on your breath and calmly saying, "I'm okay", is your grounding chord throughout the entire exercise.

Remember to focus on one memory per session. Towards the end of your session, your body will feel relaxed and your mind will be clear.

Use Stress Stopper Breathwork to release tension from the recent memory of your most Routine PTSD Reaction by following the below steps;

(t) Lie down, close your eyes, and for two minutes breathe deep and slow with your right hand on your (insert answer from (f) here) _____

_____

_____

_____

and your left hand on your (insert answer from (i) here) _____

_____

_____

_____

Once per breath, silently say, "I'm okay".

(u) Think of the memory involving (insert answer from (a) here) _____

_____

_____

_____

(v) Feel your body's reaction as you let the memory play out to a stressful moment. Then pause the memory.

(w) Imagine yourself inside that memory calmly saying, "I'm okay", once per breath, as you continually breathe deep and slow with two hands gently resting where you feel tension in your body.

Continue Step (w) for 20 minutes or until you feel the tension release from your body and from the memory. Waves of emotions will come and go. Continually focusing on your breath and calmly saying, "I'm okay", is your grounding chord throughout the entire exercise.

* Use Stress Stopper Breathwork in the same fashion to handle flashbacks. When a flashback occurs, immediately begin using the technique until physical and emotional tension releases. Focus on your breath and mantra.

Exercise 4.1 (2) Process the Trauma   **Date:** ___/___/_____

Give yourself at least 50 minutes of undisturbed space, have your team a phone call away for support, and see the process to the end.

Step 1. Routine PTSD Assessment

Assess your most frequent PTSD reaction by answering the below questions;

(a) What is the one thing that triggers your PTSD reactions most often?

_____

_____

_____

(b) Where are you when this reaction is most often triggered?

_____

_____

_____

(c) What time of day and which days of the week is this reaction most likely to occur?

_____

_____

_____

(d) Which emotion is predominant during this PTSD reaction?

_____

_____

_____

(e) What thought repeats in your head during this PTSD reaction?

_____

_____

_____

(f) Where do you feel tension right now while thinking about this reaction?

_____

_____

_____

Step 2. Repressed PTSD Assessment

Look back on your life. Identify which memory is fueling this PTSD reaction by answering the below questions;

(g) What is the 1st time you can remember thinking (insert answer from (e) here)

_____

_____

_____

and feeling (insert answer from (d) here) _____

_____

_____

_____

at the same time?

_____

_____

_____

(h) Who or what caused that previous stress reaction?

_____

_____

_____

(i) Where do you feel tension in your body while thinking about this memory?

_____

_____

_____

Step 3. Process the Trauma

Use Stress Stopper Breathwork to release tension from the traumatic memory by following the below steps;

(j) Lie down, close your eyes, and for two minutes breathe deep and slow with your right hand on your (insert answer from (f) here) _____

_____

_____

_____

and your left hand on your (insert answer from (i) here) _____

_____

_____

_____

Once per breath, silently say, "I'm okay".

(k) Think of the memory involving (insert answer from (h) here) _____

_____

_____

_____

(l) Observe your body's reaction as you let the memory play out to a stressful moment. Then pause the memory.

(m) Imagine yourself inside that memory calmly saying, "I'm okay", once per breath, as you continually breathe deep and slow with two hands gently resting where you feel tension in your body.

Continue Step (m) for 20 minutes or until you feel the tension release from your body and from the memory. Waves of emotions will come and go. Continually focusing on your breath and calmly saying, "I'm okay", is your grounding chord throughout the entire exercise.

Remember to focus on one memory per session. Towards the end of your session, your body will feel relaxed and your mind will be clear.

Use Stress Stopper Breathwork to release tension from the recent memory of your most Routine PTSD Reaction by following the below steps;

(t) Lie down, close your eyes, and for two minutes breathe deep and slow with your right hand on your (insert answer from (f) here) _____

_____

_____

_____

and your left hand on your (insert answer from (i) here) _____

_____

_____

_____

Once per breath, silently say, "I'm okay".

(u) Think of the memory involving (insert answer from (a) here) _____

_____

_____

_____

(v) Feel your body's reaction as you let the memory play out to a stressful moment. Then pause the memory.

(w) Imagine yourself inside that memory calmly saying, "I'm okay", once per breath, as you continually breathe deep and slow with two hands gently resting where you feel tension in your body.

Continue Step (w) for 20 minutes or until you feel the tension release from your body and from the memory. Waves of emotions will come and go. Continually focusing on your breath and calmly saying, "I'm okay", is your grounding chord throughout the entire exercise.

* Use Stress Stopper Breathwork in the same fashion to handle flashbacks. When a flashback occurs, immediately begin using the technique until physical and emotional tension releases. Focus on your breath and mantra.

Exercise 4.1 (3) Process the Trauma   **Date:** ___/___/_____

Give yourself at least 50 minutes of undisturbed space, have your team a phone call away for support, and see the process to the end.

Step 1. Routine PTSD Assessment

Assess your most frequent PTSD reaction by answering the below questions;

(a) What is the one thing that triggers your PTSD reactions most often?

_____

_____

_____

(b) Where are you when this reaction is most often triggered?

_____

_____

_____

(c) What time of day and which days of the week is this reaction most likely to occur?

_____

_____

_____

(d) Which emotion is predominant during this PTSD reaction?

_____

_____

_____

(e) What thought repeats in your head during this PTSD reaction?

_____

_____

_____

(f) Where do you feel tension right now while thinking about this reaction?

_____

_____

_____

Step 2. Repressed PTSD Assessment

Look back on your life. Identify which memory is fueling this PTSD reaction by answering the below questions;

(g) What is the 1st time you can remember thinking (insert answer from (e) here)

_____

_____

_____

and feeling (insert answer from (d) here) _____

_____

_____

_____

at the same time?

_____

_____

_____

(h) Who or what caused that previous stress reaction?

_____

_____

_____

(i) Where do you feel tension in your body while thinking about this memory?

_____

_____

_____

Step 3. Process the Trauma

Use Stress Stopper Breathwork to release tension from the traumatic memory by following the below steps;

(j) Lie down, close your eyes, and for two minutes breathe deep and slow with your right hand on your (insert answer from (f) here) _____

_____

_____

_____

and your left hand on your (insert answer from (i) here) _____

_____

_____

_____

Once per breath, silently say, "I'm okay".

(k) Think of the memory involving (insert answer from (h) here) _____

_____

_____

_____

(l) Observe your body's reaction as you let the memory play out to a stressful moment. Then pause the memory.

(m) Imagine yourself inside that memory calmly saying, "I'm okay", once per breath, as you continually breathe deep and slow with two hands gently resting where you feel tension in your body.

Continue Step (m) for 20 minutes or until you feel the tension release from your body and from the memory. Waves of emotions will come and go. Continually focusing on your breath and calmly saying, "I'm okay", is your grounding chord throughout the entire exercise.

Remember to focus on one memory per session. Towards the end of your session, your body will feel relaxed and your mind will be clear.

Use Stress Stopper Breathwork to release tension from the recent memory of your most Routine PTSD Reaction by following the below steps;

(t) Lie down, close your eyes, and for two minutes breathe deep and slow with your right hand on your (insert answer from (f) here) _____

_____

_____

_____

and your left hand on your (insert answer from (i) here) _____

_____

_____

_____

Once per breath, silently say, "I'm okay".

(u) Think of the memory involving (insert answer from (a) here) _____

_____

_____

_____

(v) Feel your body's reaction as you let the memory play out to a stressful moment. Then pause the memory.

(w) Imagine yourself inside that memory calmly saying, "I'm okay", once per breath, as you continually breathe deep and slow with two hands gently resting where you feel tension in your body.

Continue Step (w) for 20 minutes or until you feel the tension release from your body and from the memory. Waves of emotions will come and go. Continually focusing on your breath and calmly saying, "I'm okay", is your grounding chord throughout the entire exercise.

* Use Stress Stopper Breathwork in the same fashion to handle flashbacks. When a flashback occurs, immediately begin using the technique until physical and emotional tension releases. Focus on your breath and mantra.

Exercise 4.1 (4) Process the Trauma   **Date: ___/___/_____**

Give yourself at least 50 minutes of undisturbed space, have your team a phone call away for support, and see the process to the end.

Step 1. Routine PTSD Assessment

Assess your most frequent PTSD reaction by answering the below questions;

(a) What is the one thing that triggers your PTSD reactions most often?

_____

_____

_____

(b) Where are you when this reaction is most often triggered?

_____

_____

_____

(c) What time of day and which days of the week is this reaction most likely to occur?

_____

_____

_____

(d) Which emotion is predominant during this PTSD reaction?

_____

_____

_____

(e) What thought repeats in your head during this PTSD reaction?

_____

_____

_____

(f) Where do you feel tension right now while thinking about this reaction?

_____

_____

_____

Step 2. Repressed PTSD Assessment

Look back on your life. Identify which memory is fueling this PTSD reaction by answering the below questions;

(g) What is the 1st time you can remember thinking (insert answer from (e) here)

_____

_____

_____

and feeling (insert answer from (d) here) _____

_____

_____

_____

at the same time?

_____

_____

_____

(h) Who or what caused that previous stress reaction?

_____

_____

_____

(i) Where do you feel tension in your body while thinking about this memory?

_____

_____

_____

Step 3. Process the Trauma

Use Stress Stopper Breathwork to release tension from the traumatic memory by following the below steps;

(j) Lie down, close your eyes, and for two minutes breathe deep and slow with your right hand on your (insert answer from (f) here) _____

_____

_____

_____

and your left hand on your (insert answer from (i) here) _____

_____

_____

_____

Once per breath, silently say, "I'm okay".

(k) Think of the memory involving (insert answer from (h) here) _____

_____

_____

_____

(l) Observe your body's reaction as you let the memory play out to a stressful moment. Then pause the memory.

(m) Imagine yourself inside that memory calmly saying, "I'm okay", once per breath, as you continually breathe deep and slow with two hands gently resting where you feel tension in your body.

Continue Step (m) for 20 minutes or until you feel the tension release from your body and from the memory. Waves of emotions will come and go. Continually focusing on your breath and calmly saying, "I'm okay", is your grounding chord throughout the entire exercise.

Remember to focus on one memory per session. Towards the end of your session, your body will feel relaxed and your mind will be clear.

Use Stress Stopper Breathwork to release tension from the recent memory of your most Routine PTSD Reaction by following the below steps;

    (t) Lie down, close your eyes, and for two minutes breathe deep and slow with your right hand on your (insert answer from (f) here) _____

_____

_____

_____

        and your left hand on your (insert answer from (i) here) _____

_____

_____

_____

        Once per breath, silently say, "I'm okay".

    (u) Think of the memory involving (insert answer from (a) here) _____

_____

_____

_____

    (v) Feel your body's reaction as you let the memory play out to a stressful moment. Then pause the memory.

    (w) Imagine yourself inside that memory calmly saying, "I'm okay", once per breath, as you continually breathe deep and slow with two hands gently resting where you feel tension in your body.

Continue Step (w) for 20 minutes or until you feel the tension release from your body and from the memory. Waves of emotions will come and go. Continually focusing on your breath and calmly saying, "I'm okay", is your grounding chord throughout the entire exercise.

* Use Stress Stopper Breathwork in the same fashion to handle flashbacks. When a flashback occurs, immediately begin using the technique until physical and emotional tension releases. Focus on your breath and mantra.

Exercise 4.1 (5) Process the Trauma Date: ___/___/_____

Give yourself at least 50 minutes of undisturbed space, have your team a phone call away for support, and see the process to the end.

Step 1. Routine PTSD Assessment

Assess your most frequent PTSD reaction by answering the below questions;

(a) What is the one thing that triggers your PTSD reactions most often?

_____

_____

_____

(b) Where are you when this reaction is most often triggered?

_____

_____

_____

(c) What time of day and which days of the week is this reaction most likely to occur?

_____

_____

_____

(d) Which emotion is predominant during this PTSD reaction?

_____

_____

_____

(e) What thought repeats in your head during this PTSD reaction?

_____

_____

_____

(f) Where do you feel tension right now while thinking about this reaction?

_____

_____

_____

Step 2. Repressed PTSD Assessment

Look back on your life. Identify which memory is fueling this PTSD reaction by answering the below questions;

(g) What is the 1st time you can remember thinking (insert answer from (e) here)

_____

_____

_____

and feeling (insert answer from (d) here) _____

_____

_____

_____

at the same time?

_____

_____

_____

(h) Who or what caused that previous stress reaction?

_____

_____

_____

(i) Where do you feel tension in your body while thinking about this memory?

_____

_____

_____

Step 3. Process the Trauma

Use Stress Stopper Breathwork to release tension from the traumatic memory by following the below steps;

(j) Lie down, close your eyes, and for two minutes breathe deep and slow with your right hand on your (insert answer from (f) here) _____

_____

_____

_____

and your left hand on your (insert answer from (i) here) _____

_____

_____

_____

Once per breath, silently say, "I'm okay".

(k) Think of the memory involving (insert answer from (h) here) _____

_____

_____

_____

(l) Observe your body's reaction as you let the memory play out to a stressful moment. Then pause the memory.

(m) Imagine yourself inside that memory calmly saying, "I'm okay", once per breath, as you continually breathe deep and slow with two hands gently resting where you feel tension in your body.

Continue Step (m) for 20 minutes or until you feel the tension release from your body and from the memory. Waves of emotions will come and go. Continually focusing on your breath and calmly saying, "I'm okay", is your grounding chord throughout the entire exercise.

Remember to focus on one memory per session. Towards the end of your session, your body will feel relaxed and your mind will be clear.

Use Stress Stopper Breathwork to release tension from the recent memory of your most Routine PTSD Reaction by following the below steps;

(t) Lie down, close your eyes, and for two minutes breathe deep and slow with your right hand on your (insert answer from (f) here) _____

_____

_____

_____

and your left hand on your (insert answer from (i) here) _____

_____

_____

_____

Once per breath, silently say, "I'm okay".

(u) Think of the memory involving (insert answer from (a) here) _____

_____

_____

_____

(v) Feel your body's reaction as you let the memory play out to a stressful moment. Then pause the memory.

(w) Imagine yourself inside that memory calmly saying, "I'm okay", once per breath, as you continually breathe deep and slow with two hands gently resting where you feel tension in your body.

Continue Step (w) for 20 minutes or until you feel the tension release from your body and from the memory. Waves of emotions will come and go. Continually focusing on your breath and calmly saying, "I'm okay", is your grounding chord throughout the entire exercise.

* Use Stress Stopper Breathwork in the same fashion to handle flashbacks. When a flashback occurs, immediately begin using the technique until physical and emotional tension releases. Focus on your breath and mantra.

Exercise 4.1 (6) Process the Trauma   **Date:** ___/___/_____

Give yourself at least 50 minutes of undisturbed space, have your team a phone call away for support, and see the process to the end.

Step 1. Routine PTSD Assessment

Assess your most frequent PTSD reaction by answering the below questions;

(a) What is the one thing that triggers your PTSD reactions most often?

_____

_____

_____

(b) Where are you when this reaction is most often triggered?

_____

_____

_____

(c) What time of day and which days of the week is this reaction most likely to occur?

_____

_____

_____

(d) Which emotion is predominant during this PTSD reaction?

_____

_____

_____

(e) What thought repeats in your head during this PTSD reaction?

_____

_____

_____

(f) Where do you feel tension right now while thinking about this reaction?

_____

_____

_____

Step 2. Repressed PTSD Assessment

Look back on your life. Identify which memory is fueling this PTSD reaction by answering the below questions;

(g) What is the 1st time you can remember thinking (insert answer from (e) here)

_____

_____

_____

and feeling (insert answer from (d) here) _____

_____

_____

_____

at the same time?

_____

_____

_____

(h) Who or what caused that previous stress reaction?

_____

_____

_____

(i) Where do you feel tension in your body while thinking about this memory?

_____

_____

_____

Step 3. Process the Trauma

Use Stress Stopper Breathwork to release tension from the traumatic memory by following the below steps;

(j) Lie down, close your eyes, and for two minutes breathe deep and slow with your right hand on your (insert answer from (f) here) _____

_____

_____

_____

and your left hand on your (insert answer from (i) here) _____

_____

_____

_____

Once per breath, silently say, "I'm okay".

(k) Think of the memory involving (insert answer from (h) here) _____

_____

_____

_____

(l) Observe your body's reaction as you let the memory play out to a stressful moment. Then pause the memory.

(m) Imagine yourself inside that memory calmly saying, "I'm okay", once per breath, as you continually breathe deep and slow with two hands gently resting where you feel tension in your body.

Continue Step (m) for 20 minutes or until you feel the tension release from your body and from the memory. Waves of emotions will come and go. Continually focusing on your breath and calmly saying, "I'm okay", is your grounding chord throughout the entire exercise.

Remember to focus on one memory per session. Towards the end of your session, your body will feel relaxed and your mind will be clear.

Use Stress Stopper Breathwork to release tension from the recent memory of your most Routine PTSD Reaction by following the below steps;

(t) Lie down, close your eyes, and for two minutes breathe deep and slow with your right hand on your (insert answer from (f) here) _____

_____

_____

_____

and your left hand on your (insert answer from (i) here) _____

_____

_____

_____

Once per breath, silently say, "I'm okay".

(u) Think of the memory involving (insert answer from (a) here) _____

_____

_____

_____

(v) Feel your body's reaction as you let the memory play out to a stressful moment. Then pause the memory.

(w) Imagine yourself inside that memory calmly saying, "I'm okay", once per breath, as you continually breathe deep and slow with two hands gently resting where you feel tension in your body.

Continue Step (w) for 20 minutes or until you feel the tension release from your body and from the memory. Waves of emotions will come and go. Continually focusing on your breath and calmly saying, "I'm okay", is your grounding chord throughout the entire exercise.

* Use Stress Stopper Breathwork in the same fashion to handle flashbacks. When a flashback occurs, immediately begin using the technique until physical and emotional tension releases. Focus on your breath and mantra.

Exercise 4.1 (7) Process the Trauma   **Date:** ___/___/_____

Give yourself at least 50 minutes of undisturbed space, have your team a phone call away for support, and see the process to the end.

Step 1. Routine PTSD Assessment

Assess your most frequent PTSD reaction by answering the below questions;

(a) What is the one thing that triggers your PTSD reactions most often?

_____

_____

_____

(b) Where are you when this reaction is most often triggered?

_____

_____

_____

(c) What time of day and which days of the week is this reaction most likely to occur?

_____

_____

_____

(d) Which emotion is predominant during this PTSD reaction?

_____

_____

_____

(e) What thought repeats in your head during this PTSD reaction?

_____

_____

_____

(f) Where do you feel tension right now while thinking about this reaction?

_____

_____

_____

Step 2. Repressed PTSD Assessment

Look back on your life. Identify which memory is fueling this PTSD reaction by answering the below questions;

(g) What is the 1st time you can remember thinking (insert answer from (e) here)

_____

_____

_____

and feeling (insert answer from (d) here) _____

_____

_____

_____

at the same time?

_____

_____

_____

(h) Who or what caused that previous stress reaction?

_____

_____

_____

(i) Where do you feel tension in your body while thinking about this memory?

_____

_____

_____

Step 3. Process the Trauma

Use Stress Stopper Breathwork to release tension from the traumatic memory by following the below steps;

(j) Lie down, close your eyes, and for two minutes breathe deep and slow with your right hand on your (insert answer from (f) here) _____

_____

_____

_____

and your left hand on your (insert answer from (i) here) _____

_____

_____

_____

Once per breath, silently say, "I'm okay".

(k) Think of the memory involving (insert answer from (h) here) _____

_____

_____

_____

(l) Observe your body's reaction as you let the memory play out to a stressful moment. Then pause the memory.

(m) Imagine yourself inside that memory calmly saying, "I'm okay", once per breath, as you continually breathe deep and slow with two hands gently resting where you feel tension in your body.

Continue Step (m) for 20 minutes or until you feel the tension release from your body and from the memory. Waves of emotions will come and go. Continually focusing on your breath and calmly saying, "I'm okay", is your grounding chord throughout the entire exercise.

Remember to focus on one memory per session. Towards the end of your session, your body will feel relaxed and your mind will be clear.

Use Stress Stopper Breathwork to release tension from the recent memory of your most Routine PTSD Reaction by following the below steps;

(t) Lie down, close your eyes, and for two minutes breathe deep and slow with your right hand on your (insert answer from (f) here) _____

_____

_____

_____

and your left hand on your (insert answer from (i) here) _____

_____

_____

_____

Once per breath, silently say, "I'm okay".

(u) Think of the memory involving (insert answer from (a) here) _____

_____

_____

_____

(v) Feel your body's reaction as you let the memory play out to a stressful moment. Then pause the memory.

(w) Imagine yourself inside that memory calmly saying, "I'm okay", once per breath, as you continually breathe deep and slow with two hands gently resting where you feel tension in your body.

Continue Step (w) for 20 minutes or until you feel the tension release from your body and from the memory. Waves of emotions will come and go. Continually focusing on your breath and calmly saying, "I'm okay", is your grounding chord throughout the entire exercise.

* Use Stress Stopper Breathwork in the same fashion to handle flashbacks. When a flashback occurs, immediately begin using the technique until physical and emotional tension releases. Focus on your breath and mantra.

Exercise 4.1 (8) Process the Trauma   **Date:** ___/___/_____

Give yourself at least 50 minutes of undisturbed space, have your team a phone call away for support, and see the process to the end.

Step 1. Routine PTSD Assessment

Assess your most frequent PTSD reaction by answering the below questions;

(a) What is the one thing that triggers your PTSD reactions most often?

_____

_____

_____

(b) Where are you when this reaction is most often triggered?

_____

_____

_____

(c) What time of day and which days of the week is this reaction most likely to occur?

_____

_____

_____

(d) Which emotion is predominant during this PTSD reaction?

_____

_____

_____

(e) What thought repeats in your head during this PTSD reaction?

_____

_____

_____

(f) Where do you feel tension right now while thinking about this reaction?

_____

_____

_____

Step 2. Repressed PTSD Assessment

Look back on your life. Identify which memory is fueling this PTSD reaction by answering the below questions;

(g) What is the 1st time you can remember thinking (insert answer from (e) here)

_____

_____

_____

and feeling (insert answer from (d) here) _____

_____

_____

_____

at the same time?

_____

_____

_____

(h) Who or what caused that previous stress reaction?

_____

_____

_____

(i) Where do you feel tension in your body while thinking about this memory?

_____

_____

_____

Step 3. Process the Trauma

Use Stress Stopper Breathwork to release tension from the traumatic memory by following the below steps;

   (j) Lie down, close your eyes, and for two minutes breathe deep and slow with your right hand on your (insert answer from (f) here) _____

_____

_____

_____

and your left hand on your (insert answer from (i) here) _____

_____

_____

_____

Once per breath, silently say, "I'm okay".

   (k) Think of the memory involving (insert answer from (h) here) _____

_____

_____

_____

   (l) Observe your body's reaction as you let the memory play out to a stressful moment. Then pause the memory.

  (m) Imagine yourself inside that memory calmly saying, "I'm okay", once per breath, as you continually breathe deep and slow with two hands gently resting where you feel tension in your body.

Continue Step (m) for 20 minutes or until you feel the tension release from your body and from the memory. Waves of emotions will come and go. Continually focusing on your breath and calmly saying, "I'm okay", is your grounding chord throughout the entire exercise.

Remember to focus on one memory per session. Towards the end of your session, your body will feel relaxed and your mind will be clear.

Use Stress Stopper Breathwork to release tension from the recent memory of your most Routine PTSD Reaction by following the below steps;

(t) Lie down, close your eyes, and for two minutes breathe deep and slow with your right hand on your (insert answer from (f) here) _____

_____

_____

_____

and your left hand on your (insert answer from (i) here) _____

_____

_____

_____

Once per breath, silently say, "I'm okay".

(u) Think of the memory involving (insert answer from (a) here) _____

_____

_____

_____

(v) Feel your body's reaction as you let the memory play out to a stressful moment. Then pause the memory.

(w) Imagine yourself inside that memory calmly saying, "I'm okay", once per breath, as you continually breathe deep and slow with two hands gently resting where you feel tension in your body.

Continue Step (w) for 20 minutes or until you feel the tension release from your body and from the memory. Waves of emotions will come and go. Continually focusing on your breath and calmly saying, "I'm okay", is your grounding chord throughout the entire exercise.

* Use Stress Stopper Breathwork in the same fashion to handle flashbacks. When a flashback occurs, immediately begin using the technique until physical and emotional tension releases. Focus on your breath and mantra.

Exercise 4.1 (9) Process the Trauma   **Date: ___/___/_____**

Give yourself at least 50 minutes of undisturbed space, have your team a phone call away for support, and see the process to the end.

Step 1. Routine PTSD Assessment

Assess your most frequent PTSD reaction by answering the below questions;

(a) What is the one thing that triggers your PTSD reactions most often?

_____

_____

_____

(b) Where are you when this reaction is most often triggered?

_____

_____

_____

(c) What time of day and which days of the week is this reaction most likely to occur?

_____

_____

_____

(d) Which emotion is predominant during this PTSD reaction?

_____

_____

_____

(e) What thought repeats in your head during this PTSD reaction?

_____

_____

_____

(f) Where do you feel tension right now while thinking about this reaction?

_____

_____

_____

Step 2. Repressed PTSD Assessment

Look back on your life. Identify which memory is fueling this PTSD reaction by answering the below questions;

(g)   What is the 1st time you can remember thinking (insert answer from (e) here)

_____

_____

_____

and feeling (insert answer from (d) here) _____

_____

_____

_____

at the same time?

_____

_____

_____

(h)   Who or what caused that previous stress reaction?

_____

_____

_____

(i)   Where do you feel tension in your body while thinking about this memory?

_____

_____

_____

Step 3. Process the Trauma

Use Stress Stopper Breathwork to release tension from the traumatic memory by following the below steps;

(j) Lie down, close your eyes, and for two minutes breathe deep and slow with your right hand on your (insert answer from (f) here) _____

_____

_____

_____

and your left hand on your (insert answer from (i) here) _____

_____

_____

_____

Once per breath, silently say, "I'm okay".

(k) Think of the memory involving (insert answer from (h) here) _____

_____

_____

_____

(l) Observe your body's reaction as you let the memory play out to a stressful moment. Then pause the memory.

(m) Imagine yourself inside that memory calmly saying, "I'm okay", once per breath, as you continually breathe deep and slow with two hands gently resting where you feel tension in your body.

Continue Step (m) for 20 minutes or until you feel the tension release from your body and from the memory. Waves of emotions will come and go. Continually focusing on your breath and calmly saying, "I'm okay", is your grounding chord throughout the entire exercise.

Remember to focus on one memory per session. Towards the end of your session, your body will feel relaxed and your mind will be clear.

Use Stress Stopper Breathwork to release tension from the recent memory of your most Routine PTSD Reaction by following the below steps;

(t)   Lie down, close your eyes, and for two minutes breathe deep and slow with your right hand on your (insert answer from (f) here) _____

_____

_____

_____

and your left hand on your (insert answer from (i) here) _____

_____

_____

_____

Once per breath, silently say, "I'm okay".

(u)   Think of the memory involving (insert answer from (a) here) _____

_____

_____

_____

(v)   Feel your body's reaction as you let the memory play out to a stressful moment. Then pause the memory.

(w)   Imagine yourself inside that memory calmly saying, "I'm okay", once per breath, as you continually breathe deep and slow with two hands gently resting where you feel tension in your body.

Continue Step (w) for 20 minutes or until you feel the tension release from your body and from the memory. Waves of emotions will come and go. Continually focusing on your breath and calmly saying, "I'm okay", is your grounding chord throughout the entire exercise.

* Use Stress Stopper Breathwork in the same fashion to handle flashbacks. When a flashback occurs, immediately begin using the technique until physical and emotional tension releases. Focus on your breath and mantra.

Exercise 4.1 (10) Process the Trauma   **Date: ___/___/_____**

Give yourself at least 50 minutes of undisturbed space, have your team a phone call away for support, and see the process to the end.

Step 1. Routine PTSD Assessment

Assess your most frequent PTSD reaction by answering the below questions;

(a) What is the one thing that triggers your PTSD reactions most often?

_____

_____

_____

(b) Where are you when this reaction is most often triggered?

_____

_____

_____

(c) What time of day and which days of the week is this reaction most likely to occur?

_____

_____

_____

(d) Which emotion is predominant during this PTSD reaction?

_____

_____

_____

(e) What thought repeats in your head during this PTSD reaction?

_____

_____

_____

(f) Where do you feel tension right now while thinking about this reaction?

_____

_____

_____

Step 2. Repressed PTSD Assessment

Look back on your life. Identify which memory is fueling this PTSD reaction by answering the below questions;

(g) What is the 1ˢᵗ time you can remember thinking (insert answer from (e) here)

_____

_____

_____

and feeling (insert answer from (d) here) _____

_____

_____

_____

at the same time?

_____

_____

_____

(h) Who or what caused that previous stress reaction?

_____

_____

_____

(i) Where do you feel tension in your body while thinking about this memory?

_____

_____

_____

Step 3. Process the Trauma

Use Stress Stopper Breathwork to release tension from the traumatic memory by following the below steps;

(j) Lie down, close your eyes, and for two minutes breathe deep and slow with your right hand on your (insert answer from (f) here) _____

_____

_____

_____

and your left hand on your (insert answer from (i) here) _____

_____

_____

_____

Once per breath, silently say, "I'm okay".

(k) Think of the memory involving (insert answer from (h) here) _____

_____

_____

_____

(l) Observe your body's reaction as you let the memory play out to a stressful moment. Then pause the memory.

(m) Imagine yourself inside that memory calmly saying, "I'm okay", once per breath, as you continually breathe deep and slow with two hands gently resting where you feel tension in your body.

Continue Step (m) for 20 minutes or until you feel the tension release from your body and from the memory. Waves of emotions will come and go. Continually focusing on your breath and calmly saying, "I'm okay", is your grounding chord throughout the entire exercise.

Remember to focus on one memory per session. Towards the end of your session, your body will feel relaxed and your mind will be clear.

Use Stress Stopper Breathwork to release tension from the recent memory of your most Routine PTSD Reaction by following the below steps;

(t) Lie down, close your eyes, and for two minutes breathe deep and slow with your right hand on your (insert answer from (f) here) _____

_____

_____

_____

and your left hand on your (insert answer from (i) here) _____

_____

_____

_____

Once per breath, silently say, "I'm okay".

(u) Think of the memory involving (insert answer from (a) here) _____

_____

_____

_____

(v) Feel your body's reaction as you let the memory play out to a stressful moment. Then pause the memory.

(w) Imagine yourself inside that memory calmly saying, "I'm okay", once per breath, as you continually breathe deep and slow with two hands gently resting where you feel tension in your body.

Continue Step (w) for 20 minutes or until you feel the tension release from your body and from the memory. Waves of emotions will come and go. Continually focusing on your breath and calmly saying, "I'm okay", is your grounding chord throughout the entire exercise.

* Use Stress Stopper Breathwork in the same fashion to handle flashbacks. When a flashback occurs, immediately begin using the technique until physical and emotional tension releases. Focus on your breath and mantra.

Exercise 4.1 (11) Process the Trauma   **Date:** ___/___/_____

Give yourself at least 50 minutes of undisturbed space, have your team a phone call away for support, and see the process to the end.

Step 1. Routine PTSD Assessment

Assess your most frequent PTSD reaction by answering the below questions;

(a) What is the one thing that triggers your PTSD reactions most often?

_____

_____

_____

(b) Where are you when this reaction is most often triggered?

_____

_____

_____

(c) What time of day and which days of the week is this reaction most likely to occur?

_____

_____

_____

(d) Which emotion is predominant during this PTSD reaction?

_____

_____

_____

(e) What thought repeats in your head during this PTSD reaction?

_____

_____

_____

(f) Where do you feel tension right now while thinking about this reaction?

_____

_____

_____

Step 2. Repressed PTSD Assessment

Look back on your life. Identify which memory is fueling this PTSD reaction by answering the below questions;

(g) What is the 1st time you can remember thinking (insert answer from (e) here)

_____

_____

_____

and feeling (insert answer from (d) here) _____

_____

_____

_____

at the same time?

_____

_____

_____

(h) Who or what caused that previous stress reaction?

_____

_____

_____

(i) Where do you feel tension in your body while thinking about this memory?

_____

_____

_____

Step 3. Process the Trauma

Use Stress Stopper Breathwork to release tension from the traumatic memory by following the below steps;

(j) Lie down, close your eyes, and for two minutes breathe deep and slow with your right hand on your (insert answer from (f) here) _____

_____

_____

_____

and your left hand on your (insert answer from (i) here) _____

_____

_____

_____

Once per breath, silently say, "I'm okay".

(k) Think of the memory involving (insert answer from (h) here) _____

_____

_____

_____

(l) Observe your body's reaction as you let the memory play out to a stressful moment. Then pause the memory.

(m) Imagine yourself inside that memory calmly saying, "I'm okay", once per breath, as you continually breathe deep and slow with two hands gently resting where you feel tension in your body.

Continue Step (m) for 20 minutes or until you feel the tension release from your body and from the memory. Waves of emotions will come and go. Continually focusing on your breath and calmly saying, "I'm okay", is your grounding chord throughout the entire exercise.

Remember to focus on one memory per session. Towards the end of your session, your body will feel relaxed and your mind will be clear.

Use Stress Stopper Breathwork to release tension from the recent memory of your most Routine PTSD Reaction by following the below steps;

(t) Lie down, close your eyes, and for two minutes breathe deep and slow with your right hand on your (insert answer from (f) here) _____

_____

_____

_____

and your left hand on your (insert answer from (i) here) _____

_____

_____

_____

Once per breath, silently say, "I'm okay".

(u) Think of the memory involving (insert answer from (a) here) _____

_____

_____

_____

(v) Feel your body's reaction as you let the memory play out to a stressful moment. Then pause the memory.

(w) Imagine yourself inside that memory calmly saying, "I'm okay", once per breath, as you continually breathe deep and slow with two hands gently resting where you feel tension in your body.

Continue Step (w) for 20 minutes or until you feel the tension release from your body and from the memory. Waves of emotions will come and go. Continually focusing on your breath and calmly saying, "I'm okay", is your grounding chord throughout the entire exercise.

* Use Stress Stopper Breathwork in the same fashion to handle flashbacks. When a flashback occurs, immediately begin using the technique until physical and emotional tension releases. Focus on your breath and mantra.

Exercise 4.1 (12) Process the Trauma   **Date:** ___/___/_____

Give yourself at least 50 minutes of undisturbed space, have your team a phone call away for support, and see the process to the end.

Step 1. Routine PTSD Assessment

Assess your most frequent PTSD reaction by answering the below questions;

(a) What is the one thing that triggers your PTSD reactions most often?

_____

_____

_____

(b) Where are you when this reaction is most often triggered?

_____

_____

_____

(c) What time of day and which days of the week is this reaction most likely to occur?

_____

_____

_____

(d) Which emotion is predominant during this PTSD reaction?

_____

_____

_____

(e) What thought repeats in your head during this PTSD reaction?

_____

_____

_____

(f) Where do you feel tension right now while thinking about this reaction?

_____

_____

_____

Step 2. Repressed PTSD Assessment

Look back on your life. Identify which memory is fueling this PTSD reaction by answering the below questions;

(g) What is the 1st time you can remember thinking (insert answer from (e) here)

_____

_____

_____

and feeling (insert answer from (d) here) _____

_____

_____

_____

at the same time?

_____

_____

_____

(h) Who or what caused that previous stress reaction?

_____

_____

_____

(i) Where do you feel tension in your body while thinking about this memory?

_____

_____

_____

Step 3. Process the Trauma

Use Stress Stopper Breathwork to release tension from the traumatic memory by following the below steps;

(j) Lie down, close your eyes, and for two minutes breathe deep and slow with your right hand on your (insert answer from (f) here) _____

_____

_____

_____

and your left hand on your (insert answer from (i) here) _____

_____

_____

_____

Once per breath, silently say, "I'm okay".

(k) Think of the memory involving (insert answer from (h) here) _____

_____

_____

_____

(l) Observe your body's reaction as you let the memory play out to a stressful moment. Then pause the memory.

(m) Imagine yourself inside that memory calmly saying, "I'm okay", once per breath, as you continually breathe deep and slow with two hands gently resting where you feel tension in your body.

Continue Step (m) for 20 minutes or until you feel the tension release from your body and from the memory. Waves of emotions will come and go. Continually focusing on your breath and calmly saying, "I'm okay", is your grounding chord throughout the entire exercise.

Remember to focus on one memory per session. Towards the end of your session, your body will feel relaxed and your mind will be clear.

Use Stress Stopper Breathwork to release tension from the recent memory of your most Routine PTSD Reaction by following the below steps;

(t) Lie down, close your eyes, and for two minutes breathe deep and slow with your right hand on your (insert answer from (f) here) _____

_____

_____

_____

and your left hand on your (insert answer from (i) here) _____

_____

_____

_____

Once per breath, silently say, "I'm okay".

(u) Think of the memory involving (insert answer from (a) here) _____

_____

_____

_____

(v) Feel your body's reaction as you let the memory play out to a stressful moment. Then pause the memory.

(w) Imagine yourself inside that memory calmly saying, "I'm okay", once per breath, as you continually breathe deep and slow with two hands gently resting where you feel tension in your body.

Continue Step (w) for 20 minutes or until you feel the tension release from your body and from the memory. Waves of emotions will come and go. Continually focusing on your breath and calmly saying, "I'm okay", is your grounding chord throughout the entire exercise.

* Use Stress Stopper Breathwork in the same fashion to handle flashbacks. When a flashback occurs, immediately begin using the technique until physical and emotional tension releases. Focus on your breath and mantra.

Summary

Here we use Stress Stopper Breathwork to help process traumatic memories. This technique uses the body's natural ability to repair itself through relaxation. The more the body becomes deeply relaxed, the less it holds on to tension. While the memory is in focus, relaxation helps release tension from the memory, the psyche, and the body. The trauma is reframed with relaxation, as the body can't tell the difference between past, present, future, or what's seen in reality vs. imagined in the mind.

This is a self-care technique; something you can do on your own time and at your own pace. If you feel this tool is helping, I recommend using it once, every one to four weeks, until you are satisfied with how your stress levels have decreased. As emotions arise, just know, "it's okay". Releasing old emotions is part of the process. If tears well up, let them, express them, and continue to embrace your emotions with your breath, as you silently say, "I'm okay". Emotions come up, so we can let them go.

A memory is fully resolved when it can come to mind without triggering any physical or emotional tension in the body or mind. This transformation of subconscious trauma diminishes our automatic fear based reactions in the real world, as up to 90% of our mental processing occurs below the conscious level. In other words, this chapter is like a step stool that helps us reach deep inside all the shelves, as we clean out our closet.

"This guide is very educational. Brett's chapters take readers from understanding PTSD, through easy steps, proven techniques, and free tools that really work. I will definitely share this guide with family members who can use it. I recommend everybody read this book and download the PTSD FREE mobile app."

~ Bob Calvert, Founder, Radio Show Host,
www.TalkingWithHeroes.com and www.ThankYouforYourService.us

Chapter 5: The 3rd Key - Meditate Daily

Veterans showed a 50% reduction in PTSD symptoms after 8-weeks of meditation. (Rosenthal et al., 2011)

A meditation provides a taste of inner-peace. A meditation practice awakens the new you.

Introduction

Heart disease is the #1 killer in our country, claiming 1 person every 47 seconds. PTSD nearly doubles risk of heart disease.

A fixed time period study showed a 17% death rate for Vietnam Veterans with PTSD, and a 10% death rate for Vietnam Veterans without PTSD. (Ahmadi *et al.*, 2010)

Now, here's the good news.

Meditators have 87% less hospitalization rates than non-meditators for heart disease. (Orme-Johnson, 1987)

Do you see how important it is to meditate every day? Meditation is a lifesaver.

Setting Up Your Practice

To start, practice twice a day for 10-minutes, eventually building up to 20-minute meditations. Before each meditation;

- Use the bathroom,
- Drink some water,
- Set a timer, and
- Disable any devices that can distract you.

Below in Exercise 5.1, we see a very simple way to start meditating.

Exercise 5.1 Stress Stopper Meditation

Lay down. Close your eyes. Place your right hand on the center of your chest and your left hand on your belly button. Begin breathing deep and slow. Once per breath silently say, "I'm okay". Do your first 10-minute meditation now. Choose one meditation per week to write about in the following section called *"Meditation Notes"*. (chapter continues on page 90)

Exercise 5.1 (1) Meditation Notes   Date: ___/___/_____

What do you remember about the experience? _____

_____

_____

_____

Can you apply anything you remember to your life? If so, what? And how?

_____

_____

_____

Exercise 5.1 (2) Meditation Notes   Date: ___/___/_____

What do you remember about the experience? _____

_____

_____

_____

Can you apply anything you remember to your life? If so, what? And how?

_____

_____

_____

Exercise 5.1 (3) Meditation Notes   Date: ___/___/_____

What do you remember about the experience? _____

_____

_____

_____

Can you apply anything you remember to your life? If so, what? And how?

_____

_____

_____

Exercise 5.1 (4) Meditation Notes   Date: ___/___/_____

What do you remember about the experience? _____

_____

_____

_____

Can you apply anything you remember to your life? If so, what? And how?

_____

_____

_____

Exercise 5.1 (5) Meditation Notes   Date: ___/___/_____

What do you remember about the experience? _____

_____

_____

_____

Can you apply anything you remember to your life? If so, what? And how?

_____

_____

_____

Exercise 5.1 (6) Meditation Notes   Date: ___/___/_____

What do you remember about the experience? _____

_____

_____

_____

Can you apply anything you remember to your life? If so, what? And how?

_____

_____

_____

Exercise 5.1 (7) Meditation Notes   Date: ___/___/_____

What do you remember about the experience? _____

_____

_____

_____

Can you apply anything you remember to your life? If so, what? And how?

_____

_____

_____

Exercise 5.1 (8) Meditation Notes   Date: ___/___/_____

What do you remember about the experience? _____

_____

_____

_____

Can you apply anything you remember to your life? If so, what? And how?

_____

_____

_____

Exercise 5.1 (9) Meditation Notes   Date: ___/___/_____

What do you remember about the experience? _____

_____

_____

_____

Can you apply anything you remember to your life? If so, what? And how?

_____

_____

_____

Exercise 5.1 (10) Meditation Notes   Date: ___/___/_____

What do you remember about the experience? _____

_____

_____

_____

Can you apply anything you remember to your life? If so, what? And how?

_____

_____

_____

Exercise 5.1 (11) Meditation Notes   Date: ___/___/_____

What do you remember about the experience? _____

_____

_____

_____

Can you apply anything you remember to your life? If so, what? And how?

_____

_____

_____

Exercise 5.1 (12) Meditation Notes   Date: ___/___/_____

What do you remember about the experience? _____

_____

_____

_____

Can you apply anything you remember to your life? If so, what? And how?

_____

_____

_____

Exercise 5.1 (13) Meditation Notes   Date: ___/___/_____

What do you remember about the experience? _____

_____

_____

_____

Can you apply anything you remember to your life? If so, what? And how?

_____

_____

_____

Exercise 5.1 (14) Meditation Notes   Date: ___/___/_____

What do you remember about the experience? _____

_____

_____

_____

Can you apply anything you remember to your life? If so, what? And how?

_____

_____

_____

Exercise 5.1 (15) Meditation Notes   Date: ___/___/_____

What do you remember about the experience? _____

_____

_____

_____

Can you apply anything you remember to your life? If so, what? And how?

_____

_____

_____

Exercise 5.1 (16) Meditation Notes　　　　　　Date: __/__/____

What do you remember about the experience? _____

_____

_____

_____

Can you apply anything you remember to your life? If so, what? And how?

_____

_____

_____

Exercise 5.1 (17) Meditation Notes　　　　　　Date: __/__/____

What do you remember about the experience? _____

_____

_____

_____

Can you apply anything you remember to your life? If so, what? And how?

_____

_____

_____

Exercise 5.1 (18) Meditation Notes　　　　　　Date: __/__/____

What do you remember about the experience? _____

_____

_____

_____

Can you apply anything you remember to your life? If so, what? And how?

_____

_____

_____

Exercise 5.1 (19) Meditation Notes   Date: ___/___/_____

What do you remember about the experience? _____

_____

_____

_____

Can you apply anything you remember to your life? If so, what? And how?

_____

_____

_____

Exercise 5.1 (20) Meditation Notes   Date: ___/___/_____

What do you remember about the experience? _____

_____

_____

_____

Can you apply anything you remember to your life? If so, what? And how?

_____

_____

_____

Exercise 5.1 (21) Meditation Notes   Date: ___/___/_____

What do you remember about the experience? _____

_____

_____

_____

Can you apply anything you remember to your life? If so, what? And how?

_____

_____

_____

Exercise 5.1 (22) Meditation Notes   Date: ___/___/_____

What do you remember about the experience? _____

_____

_____

_____

Can you apply anything you remember to your life? If so, what? And how?

_____

_____

_____

Exercise 5.1 (23) Meditation Notes   Date: ___/___/_____

What do you remember about the experience? _____

_____

_____

_____

Can you apply anything you remember to your life? If so, what? And how?

_____

_____

_____

Exercise 5.1 (24) Meditation Notes   Date: ___/___/_____

What do you remember about the experience? _____

_____

_____

_____

Can you apply anything you remember to your life? If so, what? And how?

_____

_____

_____

Exercise 5.1 (25) Meditation Notes   Date: ___/___/_____

What do you remember about the experience? _____

_____

_____

_____

Can you apply anything you remember to your life? If so, what? And how?

_____

_____

_____

Exercise 5.1 (26) Meditation Notes   Date: ___/___/_____

What do you remember about the experience? _____

_____

_____

_____

Can you apply anything you remember to your life? If so, what? And how?

_____

_____

_____

Exercise 5.1 (27) Meditation Notes   Date: ___/___/_____

What do you remember about the experience? _____

_____

_____

_____

Can you apply anything you remember to your life? If so, what? And how?

_____

_____

_____

Exercise 5.1 (28) Meditation Notes　　　　　　Date: ___/___/_____

What do you remember about the experience? _____

_____

_____

_____

Can you apply anything you remember to your life? If so, what? And how?

_____

_____

_____

Exercise 5.1 (29) Meditation Notes　　　　　　Date: ___/___/_____

What do you remember about the experience? _____

_____

_____

_____

Can you apply anything you remember to your life? If so, what? And how?

_____

_____

_____

Exercise 5.1 (30) Meditation Notes　　　　　　Date: ___/___/_____

What do you remember about the experience? _____

_____

_____

_____

Can you apply anything you remember to your life? If so, what? And how?

_____

_____

_____

Exercise 5.1 (31) Meditation Notes   Date: ___/___/_____

What do you remember about the experience? _____

_____

_____

_____

Can you apply anything you remember to your life? If so, what? And how?

_____

_____

_____

Exercise 5.1 (32) Meditation Notes   Date: ___/___/_____

What do you remember about the experience? _____

_____

_____

_____

Can you apply anything you remember to your life? If so, what? And how?

_____

_____

_____

Exercise 5.1 (33) Meditation Notes   Date: ___/___/_____

What do you remember about the experience? _____

_____

_____

_____

Can you apply anything you remember to your life? If so, what? And how?

_____

_____

_____

Exercise 5.1 (34) Meditation Notes   Date: ___/___/_____

What do you remember about the experience? _____

_____

_____

_____

Can you apply anything you remember to your life? If so, what? And how?

_____

_____

_____

Exercise 5.1 (35) Meditation Notes   Date: ___/___/_____

What do you remember about the experience? _____

_____

_____

_____

Can you apply anything you remember to your life? If so, what? And how?

_____

_____

_____

Exercise 5.1 (36) Meditation Notes   Date: ___/___/_____

What do you remember about the experience? _____

_____

_____

_____

Can you apply anything you remember to your life? If so, what? And how?

_____

_____

_____

Exercise 5.1 (37) Meditation Notes   Date: ___/___/_____

What do you remember about the experience? _____

_____

_____

_____

Can you apply anything you remember to your life? If so, what? And how?

_____

_____

_____

Exercise 5.1 (38) Meditation Notes   Date: ___/___/_____

What do you remember about the experience? _____

_____

_____

_____

Can you apply anything you remember to your life? If so, what? And how?

_____

_____

_____

Exercise 5.1 (39) Meditation Notes   Date: ___/___/_____

What do you remember about the experience? _____

_____

_____

_____

Can you apply anything you remember to your life? If so, what? And how?

_____

_____

_____

Exercise 5.1 (40) Meditation Notes   Date: ___/___/_____

What do you remember about the experience? _____

_____

_____

_____

Can you apply anything you remember to your life? If so, what? And how?

_____

_____

_____

Exercise 5.1 (41) Meditation Notes   Date: ___/___/_____

What do you remember about the experience? _____

_____

_____

_____

Can you apply anything you remember to your life? If so, what? And how?

_____

_____

_____

Exercise 5.1 (42) Meditation Notes   Date: ___/___/_____

What do you remember about the experience? _____

_____

_____

_____

Can you apply anything you remember to your life? If so, what? And how?

_____

_____

_____

Exercise 5.1 (43) Meditation Notes   Date: ___/___/_____

What do you remember about the experience? _____

_____

_____

_____

Can you apply anything you remember to your life? If so, what? And how?

_____

_____

_____

Exercise 5.1 (44) Meditation Notes   Date: ___/___/_____

What do you remember about the experience? _____

_____

_____

_____

Can you apply anything you remember to your life? If so, what? And how?

_____

_____

_____

Exercise 5.1 (45) Meditation Notes   Date: ___/___/_____

What do you remember about the experience? _____

_____

_____

_____

Can you apply anything you remember to your life? If so, what? And how?

_____

_____

_____

Exercise 5.1 (46) Meditation Notes   Date: ___/___/_____

What do you remember about the experience? _____

_____

_____

_____

Can you apply anything you remember to your life? If so, what? And how?

_____

_____

_____

Exercise 5.1 (47) Meditation Notes   Date: ___/___/_____

What do you remember about the experience? _____

_____

_____

_____

Can you apply anything you remember to your life? If so, what? And how?

_____

_____

_____

Exercise 5.1 (48) Meditation Notes   Date: ___/___/_____

What do you remember about the experience? _____

_____

_____

_____

Can you apply anything you remember to your life? If so, what? And how?

_____

_____

_____

Exercise 5.1 (49) Meditation Notes   Date: ___/___/_____

What do you remember about the experience? _____

_____

_____

_____

Can you apply anything you remember to your life? If so, what? And how?

_____

_____

_____

Exercise 5.1 (50) Meditation Notes   Date: ___/___/_____

What do you remember about the experience? _____

_____

_____

_____

Can you apply anything you remember to your life? If so, what? And how?

_____

_____

_____

Exercise 5.1 (51) Meditation Notes   Date: ___/___/_____

What do you remember about the experience? _____

_____

_____

_____

Can you apply anything you remember to your life? If so, what? And how?

_____

_____

_____

Exercise 5.1 (52) Meditation Notes   Date: ___/___/_____

What do you remember about the experience? _____

_____

_____

_____

Can you apply anything you remember to your life? If so, what? And how?

_____

_____

_____

Exercise 5.1 (53) Meditation Notes   Date: ___/___/_____

What do you remember about the experience? _____

_____

_____

_____

Can you apply anything you remember to your life? If so, what? And how?

_____

_____

_____

Exercise 5.1 (54) Meditation Notes   Date: ___/___/_____

What do you remember about the experience? _____

_____

_____

_____

Can you apply anything you remember to your life? If so, what? And how?

_____

_____

_____

Trouble Shooting

When you first start meditating your mind might try to play a few tricks on you. When you sit down and begin, you may hear a few sabotaging thoughts; "this is stupid", "it's not working", "this isn't for me".

Remember, we are creatures of habit that don't like change. Your ego will try to keep things the same and your stress will try to stick with you. After 10 minutes of focusing on the meditation technique, you will win the ego battle. Your body will relax, your mind will clear, and you will begin to let go.

Here are a few exercises that can help you address the typical obstacles to a rich and rejuvenating meditation practice.

Thoughts – Recurring thoughts are a normal part of meditating. Think of them as passing clouds in the sky. When you realize you're having thoughts, *refocus* your mind on your breath. Feel the air coming in through your nose, passing through your sinuses, cooling your brain, moving down your throat, and circulating throughout your chest. As you exhale, follow your breath as it leaves your body. You can also do a little self-talk before starting your meditation, "Hey, brain, thanks for working so hard to keep me alive all these years. Right now I'm giving you a well-deserved break. I want you to stop thinking for 20 minutes. I choose to turn off my thoughts now."

Emotions – If you are feeling too emotional or stressed to meditate, take a moment to express yourself before you start. Write down or verbalize how you are feeling:

- "I feel really (enter emotion) _____ "
- "This situation with (enter stress trigger) _____ is really upsetting me."
- "I can feel the emotion in my (enter area of body where tension is) _____ "
- "I want to stop thinking (enter recurring thoughts)_____ "
- "I want to unlock and release the stress from my (enter area of body) _____ right now."

Physical tension – If you are experiencing physical tension, take a few moments to do some very light stretching and deep breathing before you start. It may be a good time to count your steps on a short walk. You can also adjust your meditative posture. Lying down or sitting with your spine and neck aligned is ideal when starting. You want to completely relax tense areas during your meditation. You can imagine air flowing through the tension, using your breath to unravel the tightness like a ball of yarn.

Tailoring Meditations

Over time you can adjust your meditation to meet your needs in the moment. For example you can change the mantra from "I'm okay" to something more suitable.

1. *For losing a loved one* - Use "I'm okay and (enter the name of your lost loved one) is okay". When someone close passes away our body worries about how to survive this situation, and our mind worries about what our loved one is experiencing. When we say, "I'm okay and (enter person's name) is okay", we are really saying "I'm okay here" and "(enter person's name) is okay there (wherever there is)". This helps us begin to reframe the loss in our mind, heart, and body.

2. *For fear* – Use "I am safe". When our cells are afraid, we must console them.

3. *For anxiety* – Use "All of my affairs are in divine order", or "All of my concerns are cared for". We may not be aware of what drives our anxiety. Calmly affirming these mantras slowly releases the feelings of anxiety.

4. *For depression* – Use "I have the power to create my life. I want to see the alive and happy me". Releasing depression can happen in phases:
   - Verbalizing your desire to be happier,
   - Imagining a vision of the happier you, and
   - Bringing that vision to life.

5. *For addictions* – Use "I have all I need. I'm good inside and out". An addiction automatically pours toxins in a deep hole in our soul, which leaves a person feeling guilty and needy. Saying this mantra while meditating regularly sends new messages to our cells and can help rewire the desire.

6. *For anger and rage* – Use "It's over. I'm okay now. I'm safe, and free to be the real me". Anger protects sadness and pain. "It's over" sends our cells the message the sadness and pain no longer need protection.

7. *For survivor's guilt* – Use "I trust, I am here for a good reason". This builds faith in a bigger picture, which is in the process of becoming reality.

8. *For a deeper spiritual experience* – Use "I am eternal".

Meditation on the Move

It's important to make a conscious effort to bring ease and flow into various aspects of your life. Identify points in your day where you tend to be more tense or stressed:

- Is there tension in your face while brushing your teeth?
- Are you worried about your day when you're taking a shower?
- Is there tension in your arms or lower back while driving your car?
- Do your hips get tight while sitting at work?
- Are you worried when you first wake up?
- Are your breaths short and shallow just before leaving the house?
- Is there a person in your life that routinely stresses you out?

If you answered yes to any of the above questions, this shows you an area in life to merge with your meditation. Use Stress Stopper Breathwork regularly throughout the day, especially during times when you realize there is tension.

The goal is becoming truly Stress Smart: regularly throughout your day realizing tension and releasing it with your breath. The deep slow breathing alone will do this, adding the touch and our mantra speeds up the process. Over time you will find your emotions balance, your mind clears, and it's much easier to navigate stressful situations.

Optimizing Meditations

After you have been meditating for a few months, you can use the following techniques for deeper relaxation.

1. Relaxing Tense Body Parts - Focus on feeling the airflow travel throughout your body. In through your nose, passing through your sinuses, cooling off your brain, moving down your throat, circulating throughout your chest, and follow the airflow back out of your body as you exhale. Imagining you can feel how cleansing the air is; cleaning your heart, lungs, throat, brain, etc. Now imagine you can direct the airflow to any tense location in your body: your neck, shoulders, lower back, etc. As you breathe, imagine directing your breath to move through the tension. Eventually, allow your breath to completely unwind the tension, as if it's a ball of yarn. Then imagine the breath cooling the area, by envisioning the color blue.

2. Relaxing Stressful Situations – When deeply relaxed in meditation, imagine a routinely stressful situation in your life. As the scene plays out, imagine you are 100% relaxed, breathing deep and slow. When you feel your body's stress trigger, pause the scene in your mind, and use Stress Stopper Breathwork to release the tension. When your body is calm again ask yourself, "What is the best way I can

respond to this situation? What's best for everyone involved?" Continue breathing deep and slow for a few moments focusing on your airflow. Maybe an idea will come to mind about a new way you can respond to the situation. Let the scene continue and see yourself *authentically responding* to the situation in a new way. This new authentic response replaces the pre-programmed re-action that was replaying over and over from the past. This technique shows your cells a new way of handling tense situations and makes it easier to change in the heat of the moment, as you've given your body a sneak preview of what you really want to do.

3. Relaxing Tense Relationships - When deeply relaxed in meditation you can imagine a routinely stressful relationship situation occurring. As the scene plays out, imagine you are 100% relaxed every step of the way. If you feel your body's stress trigger or you see the other person become stressed, recommend you both take a 5-minute breath break. Tell them, "This conversation is very important to me, so much, that I want to have it with a clear head. Is it okay with you if I step aside and breathe, and return in 5-minutes." Then imagine seeing yourself taking a slow short walk, focusing on your breathing, and returning to the situation completely calm. Imagine being able to stay calm and listen, and being able to reach common ground and a peaceful compromise.

4. Light Body Meditation – Focus on feeling the airflow travel throughout your body. In through your nose, passing through your sinuses, cooling off your brain, moving down your throat, circulating throughout your chest, and follow the airflow back out of your body as you exhale. Imagining you can feel how cleansing the air is: cleaning your heart, lungs, throat, brain, etc. Imagine you can feel billions of tiny air molecules cleansing your entire body as you breathe. After a few minutes of cultivating this feeling, give the air molecules properties of light. You can easily do this on your next inhale by imagining flipping on a light switch. Turn the lights on with your mind; imagine light flowing through the same path as your breath, cleansing your cells even deeper. Image the light fills your entire body and merges with you completely.

Summary

I have included more statistics and exercises throughout this chapter because I wanted to drive home the point of how important meditation is.

Sitting still while you are awake with your eyes closed throws a monkey wrench into your *stress cycles* as you send your body the message, "I am really okay, I don't have to worry about my survival right now. I am so safe, I can afford to sit in the environment with my eyes closed!" In truth, we can't afford not to meditate.

Meditators also showed 55% less for benign and malignant tumors, 50% less for outpatient doctor visits, and 30% less for infectious disease. (Orme-Johnson, 1987)

After a few months of practicing meditation a renewed sense of inner-peace, happiness, and genuine appreciation for life will begin to surface in surprising ways.

Meditating is the easiest thing to do in the world, because it's the only time we allow ourselves to do absolutely nothing. What's easier than that?

"Brett Cotter's chapter on mediation is a must read for any person experiencing stress, anxiety and tension. This is especially true for those individuals who are experiencing the effects of PTSD such as frequently reliving and reimagining a traumatic experience. The methods he recommends to help calm the body and mind are based upon sound principals of mediation and mindfulness and, if followed, will definitely help those who are troubled and in need. The Exercise on Tailoring Meditation, provides clear instructions for dealing with specific situations that trigger stress. I highly recommend Brett's book to anyone who wants to lower their stress, anxiety and tension."

~ James C. Petersen, Ph.D., CEO & Founder,
Stressmaster International, www.stressmaster.com

Chapter 6: Integration

Those practicing meditation for more than five years were physiologically 12 years younger than their chronological age. (Wallace et al., 1982)

Relaxation stimulates rejuvenation. Meditation is natural medication.

Introduction

The only thing needed for 100% successful integration is your commitment. Stress relief is a way of life. It's how you live and breathe 24 hours a day, not something you do for 30 minutes a day. I have included multiple integration tools in this chapter to help you integrate the 3 keys into your everyday life. These integration tools can help you prevent a future healthcare crisis, live longer, and be happier. Because daily use is so important for your future health, I have included an exercise, a *free mobile app* and a *complimentary website membership*.

Together, these tools help you develop the *Stress Awareness* of your most *Routine PTSD Reactions*. Your commitment to using these tools as directed, especially when your body becomes stressed, is the determining factor for becoming *Stress Smart*. There are also useful instructional design products that can be found at www.stressisgone.org

Exercise 6.1 Integration

Exercise 6.1 will help you remain frontloaded as to which stressors are right around the corner. It's important to be able to realistically expect stress, especially in situations where it's most likely to occur. Being surprised by stress makes it more difficult to manage. It's also crucial not to dread stressful situations; this will only manifest more stress.

A healthy middle road is being optimistic and enthusiastic to use your tools, to help you face your next stress reaction. Just imagine you are in the final round of a championship fight. You lost each round up to this point because your opponent was lightning fast, but you just noticed his left eye is swollen completely shut, and you have the best right hook in the business. It's time to take control back and these tools will help you do that. Exercise 6.1 helps you foresee stress and track transitioning triggers over time. This exercise is repeated 12 times to correlate with your 12 sessions in Exercise 4.1 in Ch. 4. (chapter continues on page 108)

Exercise 6.1 (1) Increase your Stress Awareness   Date: ___/___/_____

Refer to Chapter 4, Exercise 4.1 (1), to input your answers below. When you are finished review your answers every few weeks to make sure you stay aware of your stressors and pay close attention to your Stress Signals especially when;

1. You are dealing with (insert answer from (a) here) _____

   _____

   _____

2. You are (insert answer from (b) here) _____

   _____

   _____

3. It is (insert answer from (c) here) _____

   _____

   _____

4. You are feeling (insert answer from (d) here) _____

   _____

   _____

5. You are thinking (insert answer from (e) here) _____

   _____

   _____

6. There's tension in your (insert answer from (f) here) _____

   _____

   _____

   or (insert answer from (i) here) _____

   _____

   _____

Exercise 6.1 (2) Increase your Stress Awareness   Date: ___/___/_____

Refer to Chapter 4, Exercise 4.1 (2), to input your answers below. When you are finished review your answers every few weeks to make sure you stay aware of your stressors and pay close attention to your Stress Signals especially when;

1. You are dealing with (insert answer from (a) here) _____

_____

_____

2. You are (insert answer from (b) here) _____

_____

_____

3. It is (insert answer from (c) here) _____

_____

_____

4. You are feeling (insert answer from (d) here) _____

_____

_____

5. You are thinking (insert answer from (e) here) _____

_____

_____

6. There's tension in your (insert answer from (f) here) _____

_____

_____

or (insert answer from (i) here) _____

_____

_____

Exercise 6.1 (3) Increase your Stress Awareness   Date: ___/___/_____

Refer to Chapter 4, Exercise 4.1 (3), to input your answers below. When you are finished review your answers every few weeks to make sure you stay aware of your stressors and pay close attention to your Stress Signals especially when;

1. You are dealing with (insert answer from (a) here) _____

   _____

   _____

2. You are (insert answer from (b) here) _____

   _____

   _____

3. It is (insert answer from (c) here) _____

   _____

   _____

4. You are feeling (insert answer from (d) here) _____

   _____

   _____

5. You are thinking (insert answer from (e) here) _____

   _____

   _____

6. There's tension in your (insert answer from (f) here) _____

   _____

   _____

   or (insert answer from (i) here) _____

   _____

   _____

Exercise 6.1 (4) Increase your Stress Awareness   Date: ___/___/_____

Refer to Chapter 4, Exercise 4.1 (4), to input your answers below. When you are finished review your answers every few weeks to make sure you stay aware of your stressors and pay close attention to your Stress Signals especially when;

1. You are dealing with (insert answer from (a) here) _____

   _____

   _____

2. You are (insert answer from (b) here) _____

   _____

   _____

3. It is (insert answer from (c) here) _____

   _____

   _____

4. You are feeling (insert answer from (d) here) _____

   _____

   _____

5. You are thinking (insert answer from (e) here) _____

   _____

   _____

6. There's tension in your (insert answer from (f) here) _____

   _____

   _____

   or (insert answer from (i) here) _____

   _____

   _____

Exercise 6.1 (5) Increase your Stress Awareness   Date: ___/___/_____

Refer to Chapter 4, Exercise 4.1 (5), to input your answers below. When you are finished review your answers every few weeks to make sure you stay aware of your stressors and pay close attention to your Stress Signals especially when;

1. You are dealing with (insert answer from (a) here) _____

   _____

   _____

2. You are (insert answer from (b) here) _____

   _____

   _____

3. It is (insert answer from (c) here) _____

   _____

   _____

4. You are feeling (insert answer from (d) here) _____

   _____

   _____

5. You are thinking (insert answer from (e) here) _____

   _____

   _____

6. There's tension in your (insert answer from (f) here) _____

   _____

   _____

   or (insert answer from (i) here) _____

   _____

   _____

Exercise 6.1 (6) Increase your Stress Awareness   Date: ___/___/_____

Refer to Chapter 4, Exercise 4.1 (6), to input your answers below. When you are finished review your answers every few weeks to make sure you stay aware of your stressors and pay close attention to your Stress Signals especially when;

1. You are dealing with (insert answer from (a) here) _____

    _____

    _____

2. You are (insert answer from (b) here) _____

    _____

    _____

3. It is (insert answer from (c) here) _____

    _____

    _____

4. You are feeling (insert answer from (d) here) _____

    _____

    _____

5. You are thinking (insert answer from (e) here) _____

    _____

    _____

6. There's tension in your (insert answer from (f) here) _____

    _____

    _____

    or (insert answer from (i) here) _____

    _____

    _____

Exercise 6.1 (7) Increase your Stress Awareness   Date: ___/___/_____

Refer to Chapter 4, Exercise 4.1 (7), to input your answers below. When you are finished review your answers every few weeks to make sure you stay aware of your stressors and pay close attention to your Stress Signals especially when;

1. You are dealing with (insert answer from (a) here) _____

   _____

   _____

2. You are (insert answer from (b) here) _____

   _____

   _____

3. It is (insert answer from (c) here) _____

   _____

   _____

4. You are feeling (insert answer from (d) here) _____

   _____

   _____

5. You are thinking (insert answer from (e) here) _____

   _____

   _____

6. There's tension in your (insert answer from (f) here) _____

   _____

   _____

   or (insert answer from (i) here) _____

   _____

   _____

Exercise 6.1 (8) Increase your Stress Awareness   Date: ___/___/_____

Refer to Chapter 4, Exercise 4.1 (8), to input your answers below. When you are finished review your answers every few weeks to make sure you stay aware of your stressors and pay close attention to your Stress Signals especially when;

1. You are dealing with (insert answer from (a) here) _____

    _____

    _____

2. You are (insert answer from (b) here) _____

    _____

    _____

3. It is (insert answer from (c) here) _____

    _____

    _____

4. You are feeling (insert answer from (d) here) _____

    _____

    _____

5. You are thinking (insert answer from (e) here) _____

    _____

    _____

6. There's tension in your (insert answer from (f) here) _____

    _____

    _____

    or (insert answer from (i) here) _____

    _____

    _____

Exercise 6.1 (9) Increase your Stress Awareness   Date: ___/___/_____

Refer to Chapter 4, Exercise 4.1 (9), to input your answers below. When you are finished review your answers every few weeks to make sure you stay aware of your stressors and pay close attention to your Stress Signals especially when;

1. You are dealing with (insert answer from (a) here) _____

_____

_____

2. You are (insert answer from (b) here) _____

_____

_____

3. It is (insert answer from (c) here) _____

_____

_____

4. You are feeling (insert answer from (d) here) _____

_____

_____

5. You are thinking (insert answer from (e) here) _____

_____

_____

6. There's tension in your (insert answer from (f) here) _____

_____

_____

or (insert answer from (i) here) _____

_____

_____

Exercise 6.1 (10) Increase your Stress Awareness   Date: ___/___/_____

Refer to Chapter 4, Exercise 4.1 (10), to input your answers below. When you are finished review your answers every few weeks to make sure you stay aware of your stressors and pay close attention to your Stress Signals especially when;

1. You are dealing with (insert answer from (a) here) _____

_____

_____

2. You are (insert answer from (b) here) _____

_____

_____

3. It is (insert answer from (c) here) _____

_____

_____

4. You are feeling (insert answer from (d) here) _____

_____

_____

5. You are thinking (insert answer from (e) here) _____

_____

_____

6. There's tension in your (insert answer from (f) here) _____

_____

_____

or (insert answer from (i) here) _____

_____

_____

Exercise 6.1 (11) Increase your Stress Awareness   Date: ___/___/_____

Refer to Chapter 4, Exercise 4.1 (11), to input your answers below. When you are finished review your answers every few weeks to make sure you stay aware of your stressors and pay close attention to your Stress Signals especially when;

1. You are dealing with (insert answer from (a) here) _____

_____

_____

2. You are (insert answer from (b) here) _____

_____

_____

3. It is (insert answer from (c) here) _____

_____

_____

4. You are feeling (insert answer from (d) here) _____

_____

_____

5. You are thinking (insert answer from (e) here) _____

_____

_____

6. There's tension in your (insert answer from (f) here) _____

_____

_____

or (insert answer from (i) here) _____

_____

_____

Exercise 6.1 (12) Increase your Stress Awareness   Date: ___/___/_____

Refer to Chapter 4, Exercise 4.1 (12), to input your answers below. When you are finished review your answers every few weeks to make sure you stay aware of your stressors and pay close attention to your Stress Signals especially when;

1. You are dealing with (insert answer from (a) here) _____

   _____

   _____

2. You are (insert answer from (b) here) _____

   _____

   _____

3. It is (insert answer from (c) here) _____

   _____

   _____

4. You are feeling (insert answer from (d) here) _____

   _____

   _____

5. You are thinking (insert answer from (e) here) _____

   _____

   _____

6. There's tension in your (insert answer from (f) here) _____

   _____

   _____

   or (insert answer from (i) here) _____

   _____

   _____

Integration Technology

1ˢᵗ Key – Learn How to Stop a Stress Reaction.

- Download the *PTSD FREE* mobile app from the iTunes AppStore or the Android Marketplace.
- Touch the Stopper tab on the bottom left hand side.
- Touch the Routine PTSD button and answer the two questions.

Now your phone will send you mini-meditations three minutes before your *routine stress* starts.

- Then touch the Random PTSD button.
- Turn "ON" the Breathe Button.
- This activates the one-touch stress relief function.

Now when you touch the PTSD FREE app icon on your phone's screen you will immediately be guided through a mini-meditation to restore calmness and clarity.

You also have complimentary access to the Stress Is Gone Membership Website, which has more free tools.

- Go to www.stressisgone.org and click the Free Military Account icon at the bottom left hand side of the page.
- Click option *2 Logon.*
- Once you have signed in, then click the *Relax* button and follow the exercise.

The Stress Stopper Wallet Card is another tool that helps people learn how to shut down stress. It can be found on the products page at www.stressisgone.org

2ⁿᵈ Key – Process the Trauma.

- Open the *PTSD FREE* mobile app. Touch the Resolve tab on the bottom of your phone's screen. This tab walks you through an assessment, then guides you through two tailored meditations. The first meditation helps you release *repressed stress* from a previous traumatic memory, and the second meditation helps release tension from your *routine stress.*

The Stress Is Gone Membership Website also has tools to help you process the trauma.

- Go to www.stressisgone.org and sign in to your account at the upper right hand side of the page.
- Once you are inside the membership site, click the Resolve button and follow the exercises.

This online resource is like having a virtual yoga instructor, meditation teacher, and Stress Is Gone coach at your fingertips 24/7.

The Real-time Technique Brochure is another tool that helps people learn how to process trauma. It can be found on the products page at www.stressisgone.org

3rd Key – Meditate Daily.
- Open the *PTSD FREE* mobile app. Touch the MyMeds tab on the bottom of your phone's screen. This tab helps you configure your meditation practice, reminds you before it's time to meditate, and guides you through each meditation.

You also have complimentary access to the Stress Is Gone Membership Website, which has more tools for you to use.
- Go to www.stressisgone.org and sign in to your account at the upper right hand side of the page.
- Once you are inside the membership site, click the Relax button and you'll be meditating in seconds.

The Stress Stopper Wallet Card will also help you learn how to meditate. It can be found on the products page at www.stressisgone.org

Practice

Touch the *PTSD FREE* app icon on your phone's screen whenever you get stressed. Breathe along with the mini-meditations whenever they appear on your phone. Use the Resolve function between one and four times a month, through the mobile app or membership website. And commit to a meditation practice for at least 10 minutes twice a day. It just might save your life.

Summary

83% of people who submitted survey responses stated the *PTSD FREE* mobile app decreased their PTSD symptoms within the first week of use. Now that you have the information, it's up to you to use the tools and technique everyday. Every time you practice you take a step into freedom.

Chapter 7: Summary

This book shares the 3 Keys to Managing PTSD, which I have seen work successfully throughout my career facilitating stress relief classes and personal one-on-one coaching.

The entire program is built on a new meditation process that quickly shuts down our body's *Fight-or-Flight Reaction* by activating our body's *Relaxation Response*. This meditation process is called Stress Stopper Breathwork and is certified by The American Institute of Stress.

I have developed complimentary mobile technology to automatically sync your stressors with this new meditation process to help avert future stress-related illnesses. The book also guides you through a process to help emotionally balance the original traumatic memories that fuel PTSD. Lastly, I've included complimentary access to the Stress Is Gone Membership Website. The site tailors physical exercises and meditations to maximize your ongoing relief and aftercare.

I want you to get excited for the next time you get stressed, because now you have the tools to manage it. Each time your stress is triggered, there's a new opportunity for you to master releasing it.

Hopefully these tools will help take the edge off, just enough to make it easier to reach out, open up, and receive the right amount of help from your loved ones, support network, and counseling professionals.

I have faith you will become a pro at letting go. Good luck, God bless and thank you.

For more information go to www.stressisgone.org

"I really like how this book is written, in simple terms. Anyone dealing with PTSD symptoms can pick it up on the fly and reduce their stress. You don't have to be a social worker or clinician to use the tools and techniques."

~ Paul Sangalli, Ret. Air Force, Veterans Outreach Program Specialist, NYS Dept. of Labor

Acknowledgment

I want to acknowledge all the men and women who have been through hell and back:

- All our heroes who have fought for our freedom.

- Anyone haunted by memories and wanting to break free.

- All those who have tirelessly trained, selflessly sacrificed, fought through the indescribable horrors of combat, and have struggled returning to civilian life.

- All the brave men and women who fight with a bravery no civilian can ever understand, because they routinely face situations civilians never see.

- To all those who have chosen not to talk because they have seen the unspeakable.

As a country we must remember, they did this for us, our freedoms, so we don't have to see what they saw, so we don't have to risk what they risked, so we don't have to sacrifice what they sacrificed. As civilians, we owe each and every man and woman who served, our very best effort to make our country a better place from the inside out.

They have given their blood for this soil and it's our job to cultivate it. For ourselves and for our future.

"This guide is a unique and comprehensive approach to what is clearly an epidemic amongst our military heroes. With step-by-step logic and a hands-on approach, this important work provides a practical blueprint for veterans to use to overcome this often debilitating condition. Bravo!"

~ JR Rodrigues, Founder, JoblessWarrior.org
The Battles Are Over...Now We Fight for Jobs.

"This is an outstanding resource for Veterans that have been diagnosed with PTSD. This book includes a free mobile app and online membership. The meditations, exercises, and measurements are comprehensive and easy to apply. They have helped me personally on my path to recovery from prolonged stress as a recruiter in the United States Army. I recommend the book to other veterans!"

~ James Corona, SFC, US Army, USAREC

Glossary

American Institute of Stress: A non-profit organization founded in 1978, at the request of Dr. Hans Selye (originator of the term *stress*) to serve as a clearinghouse of all stress-related information. Today, AIS fosters intellectual discovery, creates and transmits innovative knowledge, improves human health, imparts information on stress reduction, stress in the workplace, effects of stress and provides leadership to the world on stress related topics.

Authentic Response: The ability to retain mental clarity in a stressful situation, listen to the other person's perspective, and express oneself compassionately focusing on the best interests of everyone involved.

Fight-or-Flight Reaction: A quick and unconscious neurological response to a perceived threat that stimulates defensive behavior.

PTSD: Post-Traumatic Stress Disorder, a temporary condition of high-frequency and high-intensity stress reactions stemming from the brain's venting unprocessed trauma.

Realize the Reaction: The ability to recognize that one is stressed.

Relaxation Response: A physical state of deep rest that changes the physical and emotional responses to stress. The opposite of the fight-or-flight reaction. The term was invented by Harvard Medical School Professor, Herbert Benson, M.D.

Repressed Stress: The accumulation of memories, thoughts, and emotions stemming from past stressful events that are stored unconsciously and physically inside tension in the body. Repressed Stress can be located by pinpointing where tension is experienced while a stress reaction is in progress. Repressed stress build up causes the misperception of threats and overreactions. Consciously addressing Repressed Stress can cause tension to release from the body and increase our ability to accurately perceive the environment.

Routine Stress: The stress reactions that reoccur most often in one's life. It usually has to do with work, money, personal health, a relationship, school, commute, home-life, a family member, etc. The Routine Stress details are used to surface the Repressed Stress Memories that fuel the overarching issue.

Stress: A reaction to a perception of danger, fueled by fear-based emotions, and perpetuated by worrisome thoughts.

Stress Awareness: Describes the ability to foresee and remain calm in situations that are most likely to trigger one's stress.

Stress Cycles: Refers to the details of an individual's repressed stress, such as who or what was involved in the past stressful experience, what triggered the original reaction, and how this interrelates with an individual's present day stress patterns.

Stress Signals: Signs the body, mind, and emotions send an individual, which can used to recognize that one is presently stressed.

Stress Smart: Describes the ability to: (1) realize when a stress reaction has triggered, (2) stop a stress reaction real-time, (3) surface and process repressed memories that fuel routine stress reactions, (4) meditate daily and (5) take a breath break from situations when needed.

Stress Patterns: Refers to the details describing one's routine stress such as the one thing that triggers stress most often, where and when this is most likely to occur, the emotion that is predominant during the reaction, the thought that repeats most often during the reaction, and where the tension is experienced in the body during the reaction.

Stress Stopper Breathwork: The proprietary 3-step relaxation methodology utilized by Stress Is Gone. The technique is certified by The American Institute of Stress.

TBI: Traumatic Brain Injury occurs when an external force causes brain dysfunction. This usually results from a violent blow or jolt to the head or body. Many people with TBI have PTSD, there is symptom overlap.

Transitioning Triggers: As the original traumatic memories are processed, routine stress is reduced. Over time routine stressors (or triggers), that previously caused intense PTSD reactions, begin to cause less and less stress. Eventually, the stressor no longer triggers a reaction. When this happens routine stress becomes much less, however, one must continue to be aware of new routine triggers that may arise in one's daily life.

Resources

Veterans Crisis Hotline and Online Chat www.veteranscrisisline.net 1-800-273-8255 then press 1. Professionally trained clinical staff. Can provide referral to other services, such as substance abuse treatment, marital counseling, treatment for depression and PTSD. Run by the VA. Since 2007. Over 18,000 life-saving interventions. Answered 500,000 calls.

National Suicide Prevention Lifeline
www.suicidepreventionlifeline.org
1-800-273-TALK (also chat on website).
Spanish language line 1-888-628-9454.
Funded by the U.S. Department of Health and Human Services

National Call Center for Homeless Veterans: 1-877-424-3838

The Army Wounded Soldier and Family Hotline: 1-800-984-8523

Employment
http://jobcenter.usa.gov/resources-for-veterans
https://www.ebenefits.va.gov/ebenefits/jobs
http://www.military.com/veteran-jobs

Family Assistance Programs
http://www.operationfirstresponse.org/?page_id=3640
http://www.usacares.org (800) 773-0387

Disabled Veterans Programs
http://www.dav.org/
National HQ (877) I AM A VET (877) 426-2838
Legislative HQ (202) 554-3501

Financial Resources
http://www.veteransresources.org/
http://familyofavet.com/financial_help_for_veterans.html
http://www.finaid.org/military/veterans.phtml
http://www.rspfunding.com/catalog/item/1414261/872354.htm

Outdoor Veteran Recreational Programs
www.R4alliance.org
1-855-474-2554

Assisted Living
http://www.topveterancare.com
866-704-4449

More PTSD Resources
http://ptsd.about.com/od/additionalresources/tp/OnlinePTSDResourcesVeterans.htm

http://ptsdhotline.com/

https://www.vetselfcheck.org/Welcome.cfm

http://www.familyofavet.com/ptsd_symptoms.html

www.stress.org

http://stressisgone.com/html/p-veterans.html

http://www2.va.gov/directory/guide/vetcenter_flsh.asp

http://www.ptsd.va.gov/public/understanding_ptsd/booklet.pdf

http://www.ptsd.va.gov/public/understanding_TX/booklet.pdf

www.ptsd.va.gov/public/index.asp

http://www2.va.gov/directory/guide/ptsd_flsh.asp

Related Resources
www.stressmaster.com
www.talkingwithheroes.com
www.thankyouforyourservice.us
www.strokeofluckquilting.com
www.joblesswarrior.org

Statistics

PTSD is an anxiety disorder. Anxiety disorders are the most common mental illness in the U.S., affecting 40 million adults in the United States age 18 and older (18% of U.S. population). Anxiety disorders are highly treatable, yet only about one-third of those suffering receive treatment.

Anxiety disorders cost the U.S. more than $42 billion a year, almost one-third of the country's $148 billion total mental health bill, according to "The Economic Burden of Anxiety Disorders," a study commissioned by ADAA (Greenberg *et al.*, 1999)

Post Traumatic Stress affects nearly eight million adults in America. About 10% of women develop PTSD sometime in their lives compared to approximately 4% of men. This can include people who has experienced or witnessed a life-threatening situation such as; combat veterans, victims of violent crimes and domestic abuse, disaster survivors, emergency first responders, people who have suddenly lost a loved one, children of neglect and abuse, etc. *(*Mental Health America, undated*)*

There are 23 million total military veterans living in the U.S. (U.S. Department of Veteran Affairs, 2014).

PTSD is the third most prevalent psychiatric diagnosis among veterans using the Veterans Affairs (VA) hospitals. (Ralevski *et al.,* 2014)

50% of those with PTSD do not seek treatment. (Tanielian and Jaycox, 2008)

As of September 2014, there are about 2.7 million American veterans of the Iraq and Afghanistan wars (compared to 2.6 million Vietnam veterans who fought in Vietnam; there are 8.2 million "Vietnam Era Veterans" (personnel who served anywhere during any time of the Vietnam War).

(Tanielian and Jaycox, 2008)

According to RAND, at least 20% of Iraq and Afghanistan veterans have PTSD and/or Depression. (Military counselors state that, in their opinion, the percentage of veterans with PTSD is much higher; the number climbs when combined with TBI.) (Tanielian and Jaycox, 2008)

The findings from the NVVR Study (*National Vietnam Veterans' Readjustment Study, in Four Volumes*) commissioned by the government in the 1980s initially found that for "Vietnam veterans" 15% of men had PTSD at the time of the study and 30% of men had

PTSD at some point in their life. But a 2003 re-analysis found that "contrary to the initial analysis of the NVVRS data, a large majority of Vietnam Veterans struggled with chronic PTSD symptoms, with 80% reporting recent symptoms when interviewed 20-25 years after Vietnam." (Tanielian and Jaycox, 2008)

A comprehensive analysis, published in 2014, found that for PTSD: "Among male and female soldiers aged 18 years or older returning from Iraq and Afghanistan, rates range from 9% shortly after returning from deployment to 31% a year after deployment. (Ravelski, 2014)

19% of veterans may have traumatic brain injury (TBI). (Tanielian and Jaycox, 2008)

Over 260,000 veterans from OIF and OEF so far have been diagnosed with TBI. Traumatic brain injury is much more common in the general population than previously thought: according to the CDC, over 1,700,000 Americans have a traumatic brain injury each year. (Anonymous, 2015)

7% of veterans have both post-traumatic stress disorder and traumatic brain injury. (Anonymous, 2015)

More active duty personnel died by own hand than combat in 2012. (Williams, 2012)

The suicide attempt rate for people who have had PTSD at some point is 27%, while the suicide attempt rate for the general public is 0.5%. (Centers for Disease Control and Prevention, 2013)

22 veterans commit suicide every day; one dies every 65 minutes. A recent study found that among OIF/OEF Veterans, those with PTSD symptoms were 3 times more likely to report hopelessness / suicidal thoughts than those without PTSD. Approximately 70% of veterans who have committed suicide were over the age of 50, according to a Department of Veterans Affairs study. (U.S. House of Representatives, 2008)

Studies show Vietnam Veterans with PTSD are more than twice as likely to develop heart disease, than those without PTSD. (Veterans Affairs Research Communications, 2015).

References

Ahmadi N *et al.* (2011) Post-traumatic Stress Disorder, Coronary Atherosclerosis, and Mortality. *J. Cardiology 108*(1):29-33.

Anonymous (2015) Veterans statistics: PTSD, Depression, TBI, Suicide. *Veterans and PTSD.* February 14, 2015. Web.

Centers for Disease Control and Prevention (2013) Burden of Mental Illness. http://www.cdc.gov/mentalhealth/basics/burden.htm

Cryer, B (1996) Neutralizing Workplace Stress: The Physiology of Human Performance and Organizational Effectiveness. Presented at: *Psychological Disabilities in the Workplace.* The Centre for Professional Learning. Toronto, Canada, June 12, 1996.

Greenberg *et al.* (1999) The economic burden of anxiety disorders in the 1990s. *J. Clinical Psychiatry,* 60(7):427- 435.

Mental Health America (undated) Post-Traumatic Stress Disorder. http://www.mentalhealthamerica.net/conditions/post-traumatic-stress-disorder.

Norris FH and Slone LB (2013) Understanding Research on the Epidemiology of Trauma and PTSD. *PTSD Research Quarterly 24*(2-3):1-453.

Orme-Johnson DW (1987) Medical care utilization and the Transcendental Meditation program. *Psychosomatic Medicine 49*:493-507.

Raleveski E *et al.* (2014) PTSD and comorbid AUD: a review of pharmacological and alternative treatment options. *Subst. Abuse Rehabil. 5*: 25–36.

Rosenthal JZ *et al.* (2011) Effects of Transcendental Meditation in veterans of Operation Enduring Freedom and Operation Iraqi Freedom with posttraumatic stress disorder: a pilot study. *Intl. J. of AMSUS 76*(6):626-663.

Tanielian T and Jaycox L, eds. (2008) *Invisible Wounds of War*, RAND Health and RAND National Security Research Division, Santa Monica, CA.

U.S. Department of Veterans Affairs (2014). Veteran Population http://www.va.gov/vetdata/Veteran_Population.asp.

U.S. House of Representatives (2008). The Truth about Veterans' Suicides. *Hearing Before the Committee on Veterans' Affairs*, May 6, 2008. http://www.gpo.gov/fdsys/pkg/CHRG-110hhrg43052/html/CHRG-110hhrg43052.htm.

Veterans Affairs Research Communications (2015). Study adds evidence between PTSD, heart disease. *ScienceDaily,* 26 March 2015http://www.sciencedaily.com/releases/2015/03/150326130958.htm.

Wallace RK *et al.* (1982) The effects of the Transcendental Meditation and TM-Sidhi program on the ageing process. *Intl. J. Neurosci. 16*(1):53-58.

Williams T (2012). Suicides Outpacing War Deaths for Troops. *N.Y. Times,* June 9, 2012, p. A10.

CPSIA information can be obtained
at www.ICGtesting.com
Printed in the USA
FFOW01n2031171117
43498266-42216FF